OVERLOAD

A medical journalist living in New Zealand, Jacqueline Steincamp has been widely published on health, environmental and feminist issues, and has had a long-term interest in the chronic fatigue syndrome.

Her extensive research has led her to believe that the syndrome, under its many names, may be a threat to health and happiness equal to that of AIDS.

OVERLOAD

Beating M.E.,
the Chronic Fatigue Syndrome

JACQUELINE STEINCAMP

FONTANA/Collins

NOTE

The information in this book can do much to help those suffering from the chronic fatigue syndrome to help themselves. It is important that sufferers consult their own doctors before taking any dietary or medical advice or nutritional supplements recommended here.

Each case is different. The combination of approaches found most useful for one sufferer will almost certainly differ for another.

Research, of course, is ongoing, with frequent new hypotheses and discoveries.

First published by Cape Catley Ltd, Whatamongo Bay, Queen Charlotte Sound, New Zealand in 1988

First published in 1989 by Fontana Paperbacks 8 Grafton Street, London WIX 3LA

Copyright © 1988 Jacqueline Steincamp

Diagrams by Meta Whiteside
Printed and bound in Great Britain by William Collins Sons & Co. Ltd, Glasgow

AUTHOR'S NOTE

This is a reporter's book, not a book by a medical specialist. It draws from the knowledge of many individuals in the United Kingdom, the United States and New Zealand. They include general practitioners, researchers, complementary therapists and those who are suffering from the syndrome under its many names. It has been enriched by their enthusiasm and support.

That *Overload* is seeing the light of day is thanks to Christine Cole Catley, its editor and first publisher in New Zealand. As a result of her own M.E., her experiences with sceptical doctors, and her rejection of gloomy media messages about the chronic fatigue syndrome (by whatever name), she determined to produce a book which would deal with the underlying immune dysfunction and provide a wide and eclectic coverage of helpful therapeutic approaches. She has shared with me her own knowledge and information from many contacts.

Particular thanks go to Toni Jeffreys and Jim Brook-Church of the Australian and New Zealand Myalgic Encephalomyelitis Society, whose wealth of information over the years has provided a foundation for the book. Nevertheless the ANZMES N.Z. Society (Inc), in allowing material from *Meeting-Place* and its publications to be used in this book, wishes it to be known that this does not imply that the Society necessarily approves all the emphasis and content.

Thanks are given also to Gidget Faubion, of the Chronic Epstein-Barr Association in Portland, Oregon, for her insight into the similarity of the immune dysfunction in various chronic diseases and Tom O'Connor of San Francisco, whose personal odyssey in overcoming the AIDS virus brought home to me the importance of holistic approaches in correcting immune disorders.

Others who have helped author and editor particularly are: from the United Kingdom – Dr Len McEwen, Dr Belinda Dawes, Dr Keith Mumby, Tuula Tuormaa and Patty Singleton; and from the United States – Lynn Anderson MD, Douglas Seba PhD, Reed Baker, Steve Thiry MD and Paul Stuetzer PhD; and from New

Zealand – Dr Ted Pearson, Dr Tim Ewer, Professor Campbell Murdoch, Lois Tucker PhD, Karen Guilliland SRN, Sandra Hyder and Mike Winter PhD. Special thanks go to many sufferers in all three countries. Where they have given their case histories, names have been changed.

I am also grateful to the Roy McKenzie Foundation for their grant, to Maggie Hillock of the United States Information Service in Christchurch and to librarians at the Canterbury Medical Library.

Jacqueline Steincamp
Christchurch, New Zealand.

INTRODUCTION

Those who want good health for themselves and their families must realise that responsibility for health is largely their own. Even the wisest and most sympathetic of health professionals cannot help those who do not help themselves, and there are many things that even the most sick can do, as this book makes clear.

The personal search for health for immune dysfunction sufferers will include learning, reading, sharing experiences and opening their minds to holistic approaches and concepts. It goes beyond the correction of allergies and intolerances. Self-help programmes, tailored to individual needs and to the intricate oddities of the individual immune system, mean experimentation and awareness in altering personal environment and fostering a positive interrelation of body, mind and spirit.

Those who are very ill and who have problems reading may find that the easiest first step with this book will be to study the case histories in Chapters 3, 7, 9 and 10. These show a diversity of ways in which sufferers have helped themselves and are regaining their health.

The second step may be reading Part II, Pathway to Health. This gives a brief account of medical, nutritional and other approaches to self-help and prevention, steps which will improve basic health and immunity for readers and their families. The more medically-oriented chapters in Part I will give an understanding of the extent of the problem, of what is going on in the bodies of sufferers and why certain therapies are useful.

A plan for everyday living includes learning how one's body reacts to foods and learning to avoid reactions. This will entail keeping a diary which relates foods and activities to symptoms and reactions. These should go beyond obvious physical and mental symptoms to include dreams and pulse rates.

Those who are ill will certainly benefit from joining a support group, whether for allergies, M.E., Chronic Epstein-Barr Virus or CFS. These groups address basically the same problem – immune dysfunction. They disseminate information about knowledgeable doctors and therapists, enable people to share helpful experiences and provide a supportive network for those who would otherwise suffer in isolation.

CONTENTS

How the family medical history can help in diagnosis
Diagram: Alison's Family Medical Tree

PART I
The Illness

OVERLOAD – THE VICTIMS

What does a fish know about the water in
which it swims all its life?

ALBERT EINSTEIN,
The World As I See It, 1935.

Extreme fatigue, physical and mental, is the common denominator
in the case histories of people in many countries who are succumb-
ing to an 'overload' disease unique to this century. This is the
chronic fatigue syndrome, CFS. It is a name that belies its severity
and the immune dysfunction that is its basic cause.

Among the commonest names for the illness are post-viral
syndrome, M.E. – myalgic encephalomyelitis – and CEBV –
chronic Epstein-Barr virus. Many different local names and problems of definition and diagnosis obscure the fact that this is an
illness of global significance with symptoms that seem to be
significantly increasing.

When someone's immune system becomes depressed or disordered for whatever reason – illness, trauma, environmental
insults or a combination of several factors – that person is at risk. A
chance encounter with a virus or chemicals can then trigger the
chronic fatigue syndrome.

Unlike AIDS, another immune dysfunction disease, CFS does
not kill directly, but it can shatter lives. Much can be done,
however, to hasten recovery by reducing the overload of factors that
weaken the body's defences. Nothing is simple, not even the
detection and treatment of chemical and food sensitivities. Healthy
living, exercise and a consciously balanced diet can do a great deal
to stop the illness from striking individuals who believe 'It could
never happen to me'.

These are typical examples of the chronic fatigue syndrome:

• A woman lawyer in her late 20s, plagued with a yeast infection, candida albicans overgrowth, becomes ill after using a chemical paint stripper in her London home. She is soon too weak to dry herself after a shower, too exhausted to walk up and down stairs. She cannot think of returning to work because her brain is 'like scrambled eggs'. Diagnosis: myalgic encephalomyelitis – M.E. – with a chemical trigger.

• A once-vigorous Australian farmer in his 40s is too tired, too depressed and in too much pain to move. He sits through the nights on a chair, elbows on a table, so that nothing can touch his super-sensitive upper torso. He cannot sleep so he may as well sit up. His triggers: antibiotics, arbovirus and agricultural chemicals.

• An American air hostess, too fatigued to work or to look after her San Francisco apartment, is awake all night and sleepy during the day. She puts on weight until she looks pregnant, and becomes increasingly sensitive to fumes and certain foods. Her exhaustion lasts for two years. Chronic Epstein-Barr virus – CEBV – is diagnosed, and other herpesviruses.

• A New Zealand mother, never entirely well since an attack of rubella 10 years previously in her teens, does not recover from a viral influenza. She becomes unable to read and tearful if she tries to talk for more than a few minutes. Looking after her three-year-old is impossible; her aunt moves in to help. The mother loses weight, energy and sex drive. Her usual capacity for enjoying life has gone. The trigger: Coxsackie B virus.

• A West Indian school principal in her 50s leaves Jamaica to seek specialist medical help in New York, but hospital tests and consultations reveal nothing abnormal. Her head and muscles ache, her heart pounds, her memory is impaired and she is too feeble to walk more than short distances. Her rural school is next to a sugar cane plantation, heavily sprayed. Many of the children have health problems and learning difficulties. The teacher has also been grieving for the recent death of her sister, whose child she then adopted. A clinical ecologist diagnoses CEBV and chemical poisoning.

• A young English child who enjoys school suddenly becomes too tired to get up in the mornings. He is almost too weak to walk, his limbs ache and he sleeps fitfully. His parents, both of whom are almost as ill, take turns rocking him to sleep in their arms. As a baby he suffered from colic, then 'glue ear'. The family's illhealth was triggered by agricultural chemicals and Coxsackie B virus.

These cases of the chronic fatigue syndrome are typical in that two-thirds are female, and only one person is in late middle-age. The symptoms cited, too, are in the middle range. Some people, although suffering from abnormal tiredness (which can fluctuate) and limbs that occasionally ache or have inexplicable weakness, have few other significant symptoms. Allergies or sensitivities to certain foods are common, though often unsuspected. 'Brain fog' and muddled thinking are widely reported. Other patients present symptoms far more severe and complex than those in the cases given as an introduction. CFS is an illness of degree, of symptoms that change and come and go. There are usually periods of remission.

Extreme fatigue, which may be intermittent, is the dominant expression of illness. Symptoms affecting all parts of the body and all body systems have been listed. Each person can tell of bewildering, often painful, capricious symptoms from the toes to the head, including the brain. These can emerge, one after the other, and mimic totally dissimilar conditions such as arthritis, heart disease, irritable bowel syndrome, multiple sclerosis, cancer, brain tumours and schizophrenia. Both doctors and patients are confused. Sufferers are often accused of malingering and hysteria. The number of symptoms, their severity and the path to recovery all vary widely according to individuals. Symptoms can be so severe, so endless, so unexpected, that sufferers sometimes wish they were dead. Some do commit suicide.

Many people have suffered from it, often with periods of remission, for 20 or 30 years and more. CFS appears to be increasing in severity in that initially it was thought that 80 per cent recover, 15 per cent continue with relapses and remissions, and about 5 per cent become long-term chronically ill. By 1988, two British M.E. specialists agreed that approximately 25 per cent recover slowly; 25 per cent have wide fluctuations; 25 per cent stay much the same and 25 per cent slowly get worse.[1] Accelerating research, however, offers real hope to the gravely ill.

If there seems to be a middle-class bias in the incidence, perhaps it is because the better educated are those who, in the face of malaise and medical indifference, have the resources to search out a more precise diagnosis for their mystery illness. Many have been particularly energetic people fully engaged in demanding careers who are amazed that their bodies buckle under normal stresses and appalled at their dwindling physical and mental energies.

Most victims are young to middle-aged – particularly women and people in the prime of life. The pattern of illness for children is usually quite different from that of adults, in that it is shorter and sharper with recovery that is quicker and more complete. Women up to 30 years of age often have the syndrome for up to five years. Older people may find it more difficult to shake off. Victims often have family trees studded with allergies and chronic illnesses. Their already shaky natural defences are particularly susceptible to viruses, bacteria, fungi, parasites, emotional stress, chemicals – even foods – that healthy people should be able to take in their stride.

It is a generation that some doctors describe as a new breed of people. 'The average citizen of the 1980s is biochemically and genetically different from the average citizen of the 1950s,' says Dr Allen Scott Levin, a San Francisco clinical ecologist. He believes that antibiotics, insulin, the Pill and other modern drugs, plus environmental insults, have changed the genetic and physiological makeup of those most exposed to them. 'Ordinary medical texts and training are geared to treat people who no longer exist,' he says.[2]

There are no simple explanations for the illness. The Law of Parsimony, which reduces all medical problems to single causes, single symptoms, single solutions, is totally inappropriate. Viruses, environmental toxins, internal fungi, bacteria and parasites are all involved – although not necessarily all in every case. There are no simple solutions, no magic bullets. Allopathic (Western) medicine, which generally works by targeting organs, and often suppressing the immune response along with the symptoms, is at present often unhelpful.

Moreover, diagnosis is difficult. Conventional laboratory tests are, as yet, almost irrelevant. The minor abnormalities they may pick up are by no means conclusive. The unreliability of lab tests was shown by a British diabetic researcher, who considered his debility might be M.E. He went to the trouble of having not only his blood tested, but that of his family – and the family cat. Though he was the only one with symptoms, all the family, including the cat, showed the vague signs that might indicate M.E.[3]

Searches for laboratory tests continue. In late 1988, Dr Peter Behan of Glasgow's Insitute of Neurological Studies made a preliminary announcement of his remarkable findings involving levels of Interleukin-1 Beta in M.E. sufferers (see Chapter 4).

The illness is hard to classify. As a syndrome, it is a group of signs and symptoms that occur together and are typical of a particular disorder or disease, with a cause that is usually unknown. In spite of medical literature going back to the 1940s, many doctors still consider M.E. to be 'all in the mind'. As late as 1986, the noted U.S. nutritionist and medical lawyer, Dr Victor Herbert, described M.E. as 'an imaginary disease'. He thought the best treatment for M.E. patients would be psychiatric.[4]

Anthony Komaroff, head of medicine at a Harvard Medical School teaching hospital and a leading United States CFS researcher, is convinced that the illness is real and that it is caused by abnormal immune functioning. Writing about the chronic mononucleosis syndromes, he is adamant that no matter what they are called, they represent real organic disease.

In a paper published in mid-1987, Komaroff says the symptoms are clearly organic, and many are quite severe.[5] He finds differentiation difficult, except in degree, between myalgic encephalomyelitis, the chronic viral fatigue syndrome, 'true' chronic mononucleosis, severe chronic active EBV infection, and fibrositis (primary fibromyalgia). Komaroff asks many questions about the syndromes, and says he has no answers except that he is convinced of their organic basis. In this paper, he admits to being baffled by their cause. He knows of no treatment, nor of ways to predict the outcome. He does, however, offer advice to doctors on diagnosis.

'When I see a patient without a history of chronic physical or psychiatric disease who has developed a 'flu-like' illness and thereafter (for at least six months) has had chronic fatigue and associated symptoms, I am prepared to make a provisional diagnosis – provided other causes of chronic fatigue are unlikely or have been ruled out.'[6] For Komaroff's 14 possible laboratory tests – most of which are not available to the average practitioner, see p. 218. He notes that it is 'unusual' that more than two abnormalities of the 14 listed are present in any given patient.

Research approaches have been difficult to define because of the multiplicity of symptoms, the multiplicity of apparent causes and the many names for what is basically the same immune dysfunction. As well as the chronic fatigue syndrome and the names already mentioned, these include the Icelandic disease, chronic mononucleosis syndrome, the Royal Free disease, epidemic neurasthenia, Tapanui flu, post-influenzal depression, the environmental disease, the chemical sensitivity syndrome, the yuppie plague and the Hollywood blahs. The list is long. (See Appendix I for names.) Whatever it is called, it is a syndrome which can bring human tragedy: family crises, ruined careers and financial hardship.

North American doctors and researchers focussed on what they termed the chronic viral fatigue syndrome and CEBV. As well as the Epstein-Barr virus, they studied the human B-cell lymphotropic virus (recently renamed the human herpesvirus 6 – HHV6). This retrovirus has also been discovered in the bodies of many people with AIDS. It is thought it may cause more damage than the AIDS virus itself.

British researchers concentrated on what they chose to call M.E. Dr A. Melvin Ramsay, also of Britain, took a world view of the mystery epidemics since the Royal Free outbreak in 1955, arguing that an as yet unknown virus would be found. Professor James Mowbray, of the Department of Immunology at St Mary's Hospital Medical School in London, announced in early 1988 that persistent enteroviruses (such as Coxsackie) in the gut were the cause of M.E. Dr Peter Behan originally researched persistent Coxsackie viruses as the causative agent, but by late 1988, Dr Behan had declared that M.E. can be triggered by any one of a considerable range of viruses (see Chapter 4).

The Japanese medical establishment pursued a similar disease which they called subacute myelo-optico-neuropathy. They considered it was caused by a herpesvirus possibly mutated from one which previously affected birds. Widespread epidemics of SMON have occurred in Japan since 1955.[7] However, it has now been established that SMON is not related to M.E.

By the mid-1980s all CFS researchers viewed the particular

disease they were studying as a type of immune dysfunction in which inherited, environmental, microbial, emotional and nutritional factors can combine to set various negative processes in motion. There is a growing conviction that exposure to chemicals in the environment affects susceptible individuals by weakening their immune defences, blocking nerve transmission and interfering with cell-membrane structure and function.

Determining factors for the chronic fatigue syndrome:

● **A person's genetic background**

Genes carry strengths and weaknesses which include biochemical errors at enzymatic level. Even if only one parent has genetic abnormalities, they may be passed on to the children, who may develop metabolic problems which manifest themselves as colic, croup, asthma, hayfever, hives, juvenile arthritis, etc. These are very often triggered by allergies and intolerances to foods and substances in the environment. Such people may go on to develop cancer, rheumatoid arthritis, cardio-vascular disease and other serious autoimmune problems.[8]

● **What a person eats**

Junk foods, unbalanced diets, too much refined sugars and starches all create a predisposition to allergies and metabolic upsets. This is basically because of quite marginal deficiencies of minerals, amino acids and vitamins. Such diets also encourage fungal infections in the body.

● **Soil deficiencies**

Soil and water deficiencies of trace elements, such as iodine, manganese, cobalt, chromium, selenium and magnesium, and the use of chemical fertilisers, will result in nutritionally deficient foods, with consequential hormonal and metabolic imbalances for all living things.[9]

● **Whether a person was breast-fed or bottle-fed**

Because the immune system takes time to develop and stabilise, and breast milk provides the baby with many helpful antibodies, breastfed babies are less likely to develop allergies (i.e. colic or bronchitis) and fungal infections in infancy or in later life.[10] Babies fed on cow's milk are more likely to develop intolerances to dairy products with gut damage setting them up for other sensitivities.

● **The health of the environment**
The level of nature and environmental pollution and how a person reacts to them are crucial in the development of immune-related disease. Offending substances include agricultural, industrial and everyday household chemicals – including tobacco and petrol fumes. Individuals whose bodies are laden with toxic chemicals are more likely to become multi-allergic than those whose bodies are not. Proximity to electric power lines or exposure to constant vibrations can weaken immunity. Those with vigorous immune systems are better able to withstand all sorts of chemical and environmental assaults.

● **Viral, parasitical and bacterial infections**
The immune response of people with multiple exposures to infections often becomes depressed, resulting in persistent infections. These further depress the immune system, and can have a devastating effect on the body's biochemistry.

● **Fungal infections**
Normal yeasts within the body can multiply, depressing immunity, endocrine function and many body processes, and depressing the immune response. Any depression of the immune system likewise encourages fungal overgrowth.

● **Airborne allergens such as pollen, dust, mould and fungal spores**
As well as the obvious direct allergic reactions, hormonal imbalances in women may occur at times of high pollen and mould counts, resulting in peaks of pre-menstrual problems, bleeding during pregnancy, painful periods, etc. Mould, dust and fungal spores also encourage fungal infections in the body.

● **Stress, the wear and tear of life**
Negative stresses – emotional, physical, mental, life crises, financial setbacks, accidents – all these add to the body's burden. Intangible aspects such as negative thinking and a despairing view of life itself are no recipe for physical health. Depression and

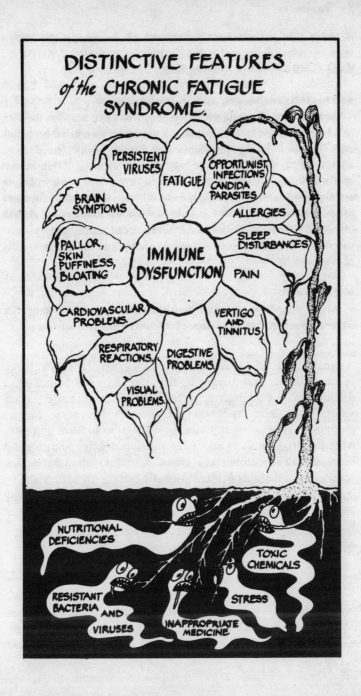

negative thinking are now recognised as depressing the body's immune response as well as the emotions. Dr Hans Selye reported these factors in his pioneering book, *The Stress of Life*.

● The Pill, antibiotics and immunisation

Women (and the children of women) who have been on the Pill, or who have taken steroid hormones to correct menstrual problems and bleeding during pregnancy or during labour, have more allergies than those who have not been so exposed.[11] Hormones and antibiotics given to farm animals to fatten them prior to killing are also implicated in chronic human illhealth and the development of resistant bacteria.[12] All these are now known to foster the growth of fungal infections in the body. Widespread immunisation campaigns are thought to produce subtle changes in natural immunity of populations.[13]

● Chance

Where people were, when they were there, and how long they were exposed to negative factors are often matters of chance or luck.

Immune-related disease does not just happen. Though a chance event or illness may trigger it, first the stage has to be set: a dysfunctioning immune system. Such disease is an active process arising from inner and outer disharmony. Its course can be profoundly affected by attitudes, by willingness to learn and grow from the experience, to take personal responsibility and to grasp every healing opportunity as it arises. A sufferer who takes up the opportunities that this particular disease offers – in understanding body, mind and spirit, and in recognising the interaction of all living things – may be able to move into a new and more rewarding way of life.

Chapter 1 THE VICTIMS

1   Dr Melvin Ramsay and Dr Betty Dowsett reporting at the 1988 Annual Conference of the U.K. Myalgic Encephalomyelitis Assn.

2   Levin, A.S., and Zellerbach, M., *The Allergy Relief Program,* Gateway Books, London, 1983.

3   Interview with author at Diabetes Conference, Christchurch, New Zealand, 1985.

4   Speaking at meeting organised by Canterbury branch, N.Z. Dietetic Assn, 10 May 1986.

5   Komaroff, A.L., 'The "Chronic Mononucleosis" Syndromes', *Hospital Practice*, 30 May 1987, pp, 71-5. Komaroff analyses differences between 'Chronic Viral Fatigue Syndrome, True Chronic Mononucleosis, Severe Chronic Active EBV Infection, Fibrositis (primary fibromyalgia) and Myalgic Encephalomyelitis'.

6   ibid.

7   Kono, R. Introductory review of subacute myelo-optico-neuropathy (SMON) and its studies done by the SMON research commission, *Japn J Med Sci and Biol* 1975; 28 (supp) 1-21.

8   Reading, C., and Meiller, R., *Relatively Speaking* explores the relationships between inherited metabolic disturbances, food intolerances, nutritional deficiencies and autoimmune disease.

9   *Empty Breadbasket? The coming challenge to America's food supply and what we can do about it; a study of the U.S. food system,* by the Cornucopia Project of the Regenerative Agriculture Association, Emmaus, Pa., Rodale Press, 1981.

10 Minchin, M., *Breast is Best* explores the role of candida and allergic responses in the mother being transmitted to the baby through breast milk.

11 Grant, E. *The Bitter Pill*, Elmtree Books, 1985. A well-referenced account of the disorders caused by oral contraceptives.

12 Lappe, M., *When Antibiotics Fail: reinforcing the human ecology*, North Atlantic Books, Berkeley, 1986, p.xviii.

13 Buttram, H.E. and Hoffman, J.C., 'Vaccinations and Immune Malfunction', *Mothering*, Summer 1983, pp 36-9.

ENVIRONMENT AND HEALTH

> The most alarming of all man's assaults upon
> the environment is the contamination of air,
> earth, rivers and sea with dangerous and even
> lethal material. This pollution is for the most
> part irrecoverable; the chain of evil it initiates
> not only in the world that must support life but
> in living tissues is for the most part irreversible.
>
> RACHEL CARSON, *Silent Spring*, 1962.

The environment of today has sinister differences from that of our
ancestors – even that of our immediate forebears, our parents and
grandparents. Few realise how much environmental quality has
deteriorated in the past 40 yeas, how fast it deteriorates day by day.
Climatic disasters are regularly in the news: floods, mudslides,
droughts, heatwaves, record-breaking snowstorms, and hurricanes
where hurricanes never happened before. News reports bring daily
accounts of killer smogs, acid rain, the growing hole in the ozone
layer, atmospheric carbon-dioxide build-up, major chemical spills,
environmental illness, human poisonings and species under threat.
As a single instance, on 1 June 1988 newspapers in the West
reported hundreds of seals dying from virus-triggered immune
dysfunction caused by pollution in the North Sea, with all marine
life off the Norwegian coast threatened by a 100-kilometre long and
20-kilometre wide carpet of algae nourished by agricultural chemicals. The virus, at first thought to be avian herpes, was later
diagnosed as the morbilli virus, related to canine distemper. It is
now thought to be an entirely new virus.

A quarter of a century after Rachel Carson's prophetic study of
man's destruction of nature, every warning in *Silent Spring* is

coming true.

The facts are horrifying but acknowledging them is of course the first step towards change.

Since World War I, and certainly since the 1950s, the world has been increasingly exposed to toxic chemicals, electromagnetic radiation and radioactive fallout. Carson wrote in 1962 that almost 500 new chemicals appeared every year in the United States alone. 'The figure is staggering and its implications are not easily grasped – five hundred new chemicals to which the bodies of men and animals are required somehow to adapt each year, chemicals totally outside the limits of biologic experience.'[1] In 1985, about 6,000 new chemicals **each week** were registered in the United States alone.[2] In the space of little more than 40 years, an overload of agricultural chemicals, petroleum-based plastics, atomic radiation, antibiotics, oral contraceptives, denatured foods and chemical food additives have become integral to the human experience.

Crucial to the overload, both external and internal, is the population explosion, with its accompanying stress on all ecosystems. In 1650, the world's population was an estimated 508 million. In 1950, it was 2,516 billion. By the year 2000, it is expected to reach 6,514 billion. As numbers increase, so do levels of pollution build up in air, soil and water. Chlorofluorocarbons and emissions from many millions of motor vehicles and high altitude jet planes are weakening the protective ozone layer, thus increasing immune damage from ultraviolet light. Carbon dioxide from burning fossil fuels is warming the atmosphere to create the 'greenhouse effect'. Sulphur dioxide and nitrous oxides are combining in the air to form acid rain which is particularly affecting northern hemisphere forests. Forest denudation is reducing the world's protection against the increasing climatic instability. Yet the eyes of most of the world's leaders remain fixed on military superiority; on missile and nuclear testing on earth and in space.

The stresses on living things increase as resistance to chemicals builds up in pathogens. Only seven insects were considered resistant to pesticides in 1940. By 1986, after billions of dollars spent on pesticides and millions of tonnes of toxic chemicals had been spread around the world, 477 insects were resistant, with 20 totally immune to any known pesticide. It is now difficult for chemically-oriented farmers to meet production targets without an ever-increasing expenditure on pesticides to combat disease, pests and weeds. It is difficult for doctors and veterinarians to cure infections witout large quantities of antibiotics. There is widespread evidence to show that, because of the chemical loads they carry, plants, animals and humans are more susceptible to disease, and especially to chronic, systemic diseases. Suddenly, within just the past 40 years, a blink of an eye in the history of the world, it is becoming very difficult for all living things. Yet the usual response is to use yet more chemicals and more drugs rather than to obey the laws of nature.

By 1984 it was estimated that pesticides (many of which are banned by the countries in which they are manufactured) kill about 10,000 people every year in developing countries, and an estimated total of 375,000 are poisoned by them. The British Soil Association, in its *Pall of Poison*[3] report, says of chemical residues: 'Their presence in the air we breathe as a by-product of chemical farming is a major scandal which must be ended with urgency. It could explain many of the diseases and deformities to which our population becomes prey. Cancers, multiple sclerosis, allergies, asthma and the like – what links may these scourges have with the growing contamination of our atmosphere?'

The world has an image of nuclear-free New Zealand as an unpolluted country. Yet, with a population of only 3.25 million, it spends around NZ$100m yearly on agricultural chemicals, up from NZ$450,000 in 1952. It was the last country in the world to continue manufacturing 2,4,5-T. Some agricultural land is so saturated with chemicals, and particularly DDT, that farmers are unable to 'go organic'. The use of organophosphates and other types of agricultural pesticides and herbicides is widespread in rural areas and is popularly believed to be associated with high rates of chronic diseases and myalgic encephalomyelitis or 'Tapanui 'flu', the common New Zealand term for the chronic fatigue syndrome.

HUMAN HEALTH

For every person suffering from an illness coming under the umbrella of the chronic fatigue syndrome who has been diagnosed and recorded, there are hundreds of thousands of people for whom their illhealth is a nameless and unrecognised malaise. CFS appeared formerly in epidemics, as well as in sporadic cases. It now appears to be endemic. As the incidence has become more widespread, sporadic cases have an epidemic frequency, and beleaguered health authorities, unable to cope or cure, are inclined to downgrade both its incidence and its severity.

Although medical libraries contain many articles about and references to CFS under its many names, doctors on the whole have still not come to grips with it. This may be partly because the illness does not end lives as does the acquired immune deficiency syndrome, AIDS. The facts that levels of immune dysfunction experienced in CFS can shatter lives and that it may lead on to serious disease are still not generally appreciated by the medical profession.

The rural Nevada GPs and now leading CFS researchers, Dr Paul Cheney and his partner Dr Dan Peterson, turned the attention of Americans to the chronic fatigue syndrome epidemic at Lake Tahoe, Nevada, in 1985. Cheney summed up the situation at a Portland, Oregon, conference on Chronic Epstein-Barr Virus in November 1987. 'Governments have a major crisis, AIDS, on their hands. The recognition that there is another viral immune-altering disease is totally unacceptable to them at the present time.'

AIDS is already stretching health budgets around the world. Virtually nothing has been spent on CFS. Health advisers to governments explain this away by saying that no universally applicable diagnoses and acceptable definitions are available. A common pattern has been denial: denial by the bulk of the medical profession that M.E. or CEBV (or whatever the local name) is anything more than depression following a viral 'flu; and denial that the illness is part of a growing world pattern. Fifty-four years after the 1934 Los Angeles outbreak, American researchers were on the verge of agreeing on a universally applicable name – the chronic fatigue and immune dysfunction syndrome – CFIDS. This name is now being used by a number of United States support groups.

The conservative elements within the United States medical establishment, such as the Centers for Disease Control, overrode them with the less threatening and less accurate 'chronic fatigue syndrome'. This is unfortunate, to say the least. Their thinking is outlined in a paper in *Annals of Internal Medicine*, March 1988. Entitled 'Chronic Fatigue Syndrome, a working definition', it completely overlooks changes that take place throughout the immune system.[4]

Ever-increasing media attention, prompted by individual vocal sufferers, is bringing the situation to public (hence professional) notice. The momentum of lobbying and research has resulted in the World Health Organisation making the illness one of the main agenda items for its November 1988 meeting in Rome. Letterwriting campaigns organised by various American support groups have also resulted in Congress approving $1m for a research programme at the Atlanta Disease Center, instruction to the National Institutes of Health for more research, and a much needed surveillance network to monitor the incidence. In Britain in 1988, a Scottish Member of Parliament, Mr Jimmy Hood, was given leave to present a bill requiring an annual report to Parliament on the incidence of M.E. and research being carried out.

Its incidence is unknown. Sporadic cases of CFS (under its many names), are not yet listed in the health records of any country, although obvious epidemics are usually noted. Steps are now afoot in both the United States and the United Kingdom for annual reports of incidence. The most significant estimate of its prevalence in 1987 was given by Dr Anthony Komaroff in a report[5] on associated health problems of all outpatients at a Harvard Medical School teaching hospital. One-fifth had suffered CFS-type symptoms for at least six months – severe fatigue with chronic sore throat, aching muscles, body pains and headache. Some had been bedridden for periods. By 1987, it was estimated that there might be as many as 300,000 people affected in the United Kingdom. In the United States, a number of similar but differently named chronic viral syndromes and environmental diseases accounted for some hundreds of thousands, if accumulated newspaper reports can be believed.

Medical journals carry more reports of epidemics in the United Kingdom and the United States together than in all other countries. Unlike the somewhat similar multiple sclerosis, CFS is not confined to temperate climates. Epidemic outbreaks have occurred from Sierra Leone to Australia, in Japan, the Soviet Union's Pacific coast, Greece, New Zealand, Scotland.

Poliomyelitis appeared to be closely linked with early outbreaks. The first recorded epidemic of CFS occurred in Los Angeles hospitals in 1934, appearing a few weeks after a poliomyelitis outbreak. Those most affected were young nurses. It was first thought to be the aftermath of polio, but the disease process took a different course. Six months after the outbreak, 55 per cent of those affected were still ill. Another 300 sporadic cases were recorded in Southern California between 1948 and 1965. In 1987, Cheney estimated 105,000 cases in Los Angeles alone, and predicted 12 million cases within the next few years.[6]

An epidemic in 1948-9 in Iceland gained the syndrome the name 'Icelandic Disease'. It too followed a small outbreak of polio and was first diagnosed as such. There were 465 cases in the town of Akureyi (6.7 per cent of the population). The highest incidence occurred in the 15-19 age group. A nearly two-thirds higher incidence occurred among adult females than among adult males. The New York Department of Health and the Johns Hopkins University School of Hygiene and Public Health carried out extensive laboratory testing of blood specimens from the Icelandic patients. No virus was discovered.[7] More than half those affected were still unwell by 1955. 'A previously unrecognised infection has persisted in various parts of the world during the past seven years,' was the conclusion of the Icelandic medical researchers in their 1955 follow-up study.[8] It was suggested that the new disease somehow suppressed the process of poliomyelitis since none of those affected in the Icelandic outbreaks contracted polio. This apparent polio-suppression has been noted elsewhere.

Poliomyelitis preceded a further Icelandic epidemic in 1955, and one in Adelaide, Australia, in 1951. This affected more than 1,000 people.[9] No specific cause was found for the latter.

Small hospital-based epidemics occurred in Britain in 1952 and 1953. The famous outbreak of myalgic encephalomyelitis, M.E., among medical and nursing staff at the Royal Free Hospital in Hampstead, London, in 1955 overshadowed an epidemic that year in Cumbria[10] and a steady trickle of cases from all over London between 1955 and 1958. Altogether, 292 Royal Free staff members became ill with M.E., firstly young nurses, then older staff.

The major report on the Royal Free epidemic and its 292 victims was made by Dr A. Melvin Ramsay.[11] He excluded from his report 92 nurses who had thought themselves to be ill, but who were later found not to be M.E. sufferers. These nurses, observing so many of their colleagues stricken with M.E., and stressed by their own extra workloads, perhaps not unnaturally believed themselves to be developing similar symptoms. The epithet of 'mass hysteria' was later applied to this whole epidemic when two psychiatrists, McEvedy and Beard, made a psychiatric assessment[12] of the symptoms reported by the 92 nurses excluded from the Ramsay report. This study, which declared that M.E. was psychosomatic, was extensively publicised and gained greater credence than Dr Ramsay's original report. The McEvedy and Beard study is important because of the great bearing it has had on worldwide medical perceptions of the condition. Most doctors have for years regarded 'the Royal Free Disease' as a dustbin condition or a refuge for hypochondriacs. There has been difficulty in recognising that no matter what it is called, CFS is indeed a disease, with specific disease processes and a confusing syndrome of symptoms.

Events have at last vindicated Dr Ramsay and his long championship of victims of the Royal Free and similar epidemics. His book, *Postviral Fatigue Syndrome: the Saga of Royal Free Disease*, was published in 1987.[13]

Widespread outbreaks of CFS in the 1960s and 1970s in Northern England and Scotland were thought to be caused primarily by the Coxsackie B virus. The Echo 9 virus was implicated in a Lancashire outbreak in 1959[14] and the Echo 19 virus was implicated in Birmingham in 1975.[15] CFS now appears to be endemic in the United Kingdom, particularly on the west coast of Scotland. An association was set up for British sufferers in 1980 with Dr Ramsay as president. (See Contact Addresses of Support and Action Groups on page 222.)

In Australia, epidemics have occurred with increasing frequency since a 1976 outbreak in Sydney. A widespread CFS epidemic in Southern Queensland in 1980-81 was thought to be triggered by the herbicides 2,4-D and 2,4,5-T.[16] This was followed by a 1984 epidemic in the northern New South Wales town of Gunnedah, where 1000 people fell ill. Studies showed that body levels of antibiotics and agricultural chemicals were crucial in determining the victims. The same levels of the virus responsible were also measured in healthy people in neighbouring unsprayed areas. The virus plus the antibiotics appeared to upset homeostasis (the natural balance and functioning) of the bodies of sensitive persons so that they developed hypersensitive reactions to the agricultural chemicals.[17]

Sensational news stories about CFS now appear regularly in the United States. A number of causes are recognised, from environmental insults to any of several viruses. After many small outbreaks across the nation, often with differing 'discovered' causes, there was a major epidemic in New York in 1984 triggered by the Epstein-Barr virus (one of the herpes family and associated with glandular fever). The condition became popularly known as CEBV, Chronic Epstein-Barr virus. By 1987, there were more than 200 American support groups for those suffering from CEBV and persistent viruses. In mid-1988, the figure had risen to 320.

Most attention focussed on an outbreak at the Nevadan resort town, Incline Village, at Lake Tahoe. It began quietly in 1984, but two years later serious neurological damage and problems in thinking (cognitive dysfunction) were showing up in many of those affected. By 1988, brain changes similar to those in multiple sclerosis and AIDS, and normally rare T cell and B cell cancers, were found in a few Lake Tahoe cases.

As a result of the determination and inquiring minds of Lake Tahoe doctors Cheney and Peterson, major breakthroughs were made into the nature of CFS. Leading virologists and medical researchers such as Dr Robert Gallo, co-discoverer of the AIDS virus, and Dr Anthony Komaroff became interested in the disease. The human B cell lymphotropic virus (HBLV) was isolated in many Lake Tahoe blood samples. HBLV is a member of the herpes family, like EBV, and is the first herpesvirus discovered since 1967.

A New Zealander who became ill in the 1976 Sydney M.E. epidemic wrote what is believed to be the first book on the syndrome. Published in 1982, *The Mile-High Staircase* is by Toni Jeffreys.[18] She and her husband Jim Brook-Church founded the Australian and New Zealand Myalgic Encephalomyelitis Society, ANZMES, in 1980.

A major New Zealand outbreak of CFS occurred in 1983 in the little Otago township of Tapanui.[19] It was brought to the attention of New Zealanders by the efforts of a local GP, Dr Peter Snow, who recognised the epidemic's unusual dimensions.[20] It appeared to be triggered by an Asian 'flu epidemic which involved the Coxsackie B virus. The popular term 'Tapanui 'flu' helped to obscure the severity of the condition. Whole families were stricken and about a sixth of the population was affected. Tapanui is the centre of a rural area which has one of New Zealand's highest incidences of cot deaths and multiple sclerosis, and high levels of arthritis and asthma. Cases then occurred with increasing frequency throughout New Zealand until it seemed that most people knew of sufferers. In 1988, the New Zealand Health Department held an 'M.E. Awareness Week'.

Understanding CFS is not easy. The chapters ahead may present challenges. As Jay Goldstein, psychoneuroimmunologist at the University of California's Irvine campus, says: 'To me, this is the most complex disease in all of medicine because there are so many variables. It makes some people wonder if the way it works is beyond the capacity of the human brain to understand.'[21]

RECOMMENDED READING:

Silent Spring, by Rachel Carson, Hamish Hamilton, U.K., 1962.
High Tech Holocaust, by James Bellini, Greenhouse Publications Pty Ltd, Australia, 1987.
Modern Meat: Antibiotics, Hormones and the Pharmaceutical Farm, by Orville Schell, Vintage Books, U.S., 1985.
Agricide: The Hidden Crisis that Affects Us All, by Dr Michael W. Fox, Schocken Books, U.S., 1986.
The Mile-High Staircase, by Toni Jeffreys, Hodder & Stoughton, U.K., 1982. The story of her own illness.
Acid Earth: The global threat of acid pollution, by John McCormick, International Institute for Environment and Development, London, 1985.

Chapter 2   ENVIRONMENT AND HEALTH

1   Carson, R, *Silent Spring*, Hamish Hamilton, 1962, p.6.
2   Gard, Z.R., et al., 'The Bio-Toxic Reduction Program: Eliminating "Body" Pollution', *Townsend Letter for Doctors*, Apr 1987; 46: 49-59.
3   British Soil Association, *Pall of Poison* report, 1984.
4   Holmes, G.P., et al., 'Chronic Viral Fatigue: A Working Case Definition', *Annals of Internal Medicine*, 108, 3, March 1988, pp. 387-9.

5   Komaroff, A., *Jnl American Med. Assn.*, 1 May 1987.
6   Johnson, H., 'Journey into Fear: the growing nightmare of EBV', *Rolling Stone*, two parts, 30 July and 1 August 1987.
7   Sigurdsson, B., et al., 'A disease epidemic in Iceland resembling poliomyelitis', *Am Jnl Hygiene*, 52, 222, 1950.
8   Sigurdsson, B., et al., 'Clinical findings six years after outbreak of Akureyi Disease', *Lancet*, 1, 766.
9   Pellew, R.A.A., et al., 'Further Investigations on a disease resembling poliomyelitis seen in Adelaide', *Med Jnl Aust.*, 42 ii, 480, 1955.
10 Wallis, A.L., 'An unusual epidemic', *Lancet*, 1955 ii 1091.
11 Ramsay, A.M., 'Encephalomyelitis in North West London; an endemic infection simulating poliomyelitis and hysteria', *Lancet*, 1970; i: 969-71.
12 McEvedy, C.P. and Beard, A.W., 'Royal Free Epidemic of 1955; a reconsideration', *BMJ*, 1, 7, 1970.
13 Ramsay, A.M., *Postviral Fatigue Syndrome: the Saga of Royal Free Disease*, Gower Medical for the Myalgic Encephalomyelitis Association, 1986.
14 Lyle, W.H., 'An outbreak of disease believed to have been caused by Echo 9 virus', *Annals of Internal Medicine*, 51, 248, 1959.
15 Bali, A.F., 'Disease due to Echovirus Type 19 in Birmingham, England, 1975: relationship to epidemic neurasthenia', in Epidemic Neuromyasthenia 1934-1978: Current Approaches, Symposium, Royal Society of Medicine, London, 1978. *Post-Graduate Medical Journal*, 54, pp. 737-40.
16 Steincamp, J. 'Living with an Agent Orange Cocktail', *National Times*, Sydney, 18 Jan 1981.
17 'Town stricken by mysterious disease', *The Australian*, 6 February 1984.
18 Jeffreys, T., *The Mile-High Staircase*, Hodder & Stoughton, 1982.
19 Steincamp, J., 'M.E. – mystery epidemic', *N.Z. Listener*, 19 May 1984.
20 Poore, M., Snow, P. and Paul, C., 'An Unexplained Illness in West Otago', *N.Z. Medical Journal*, 13 June 1984, 97:757.
21 Goldstein, J., interview in *Santa Fe Reporter*, 3 March 1988.

CASE HISTORIES:
TWO WOMEN

The stories of two women, who became ill at about the same time at opposite sides of the world, illustrate many of the points already made in this book.

Neither was as severely affected as some whose case histories appear later, but both had to persevere in the face of early medical disbelief until a diagnosis and appropriate treatment were forthcoming. Although there were many differences in their symptoms, both women were ill for nearly four years. Both believe they have now recovered.

KATE

Kate's story is international. She became ill in New Zealand, recovered somewhat while travelling through Africa, then relapsed in England. She went to India where the hot dry climate, like Africa's, again made her feel slightly better. Once back in London she became very ill indeed but there she was eventually found to have M.E. (Coxsackie B virus) and began the road to recovery. On her way back to New Zealand, Kate says, she found support groups in the United States to be particularly helpful. She is a writer in her 60s.

'I became ill in 1984 with what I thought was influenza – a 'flu which wouldn't go away. I haven't met anyone as old as I was when the chronic fatigue and immune dysfunction syndrome first struck, though I've heard of a surgeon aged 72 who was able to play squash again when he was 75.

'The cheerful fact in my case is that I think I have now recovered, but this took a lot of work and, I suspect, a lot of luck.'

Kate was spending a weekend as a guest on a Maori marae when she became ill. The Maori form of greeting, the hongi, involves nose to nose contact and the respectful inhalation of the other's breath. Many Maoris and Europeans became ill with influenza after that weekend, but to Kate's knowledge she was the only person who did not recover in the usual time.

'I certainly didn't know this then – in fact it took me two years of miserable searching to discover what was happening – but I know now that my immune system was dysfunctioning and I was ripe and ready to be tipped into chronic illness. It's important for everyone to have some idea of what can damage their immune systems, as this is an area where people can take special care, so I should say what had happened to me.

'Intense grief after my husband's death had sent me spiralling down into a state where I seemed barely functioning. Sooner or later grief touches nearly everyone, so we should know – I didn't – what physical effects grief can have, and what one can do to try to build up one's immune system. If I had found someone knowledgeable to help me with the extra vitamins and minerals my body obviously needed then, I wouldn't have got at such a low ebb physically as well as emotionally.

'Then, when I was beginning to feel that one day I could be a whole and healthy person again, I decided this was the time to make yet another heroic effort to stop smoking. For me it was indeed heroic. I had tried hard, so often, to stop but I was smoking some 50 cigarettes a day, smoking as if my life depended on the habit. And my life – as I lived it – did. Millions of words published or broadcast – and all were irrevocably associated with smoking cigarettes. When at last I managed to stop (aided by friends who stopped smoking at the same time, and by Nicorettes and the tricyclic, Sinequan) I felt pole-axed to the last fibre of my being. Certainly I had begun to be less likely a candidate for emphysema or lung cancer, but this second shock obviously didn't spare my immune system.'

Kate believes everyone should be aware of the crises which affect immune systems – 'Our grandmothers used to talk about the dangers of being run down, or having a low resistance' – and the need to be specially careful at such times. She says her previous good health had led her to shrug off such concerns.

When her illness struck, she had eight months in which to finish researching and writing two promised books, time and to spare had she been able to work normally. But she felt overwhelmed by a peculiar fatigue, 'as if I were trying to walk under water. Every sentence seemed to have to be dragged out of me, by pincers.'

Tests by her GP revealed nothing. All systems were apparently normal. She looked much the same as usual except that she began to put on weight, 'a kind of puffiness'. Her GP treated intensely painful attacks of sore throat with antibiotics.

She received no treatment for her next misadventure – eating a bowl of salad greens affected by the chemical 2,4,5-T – as she didn't discover until much later that a vegetable supply had been contaminated by this poison, and she had no way of knowing how much of the diluted chemical had been ingested.

Kate then heard of others stricken with extraordinary fatigue, among them several New Zealand writers and publishers. 'I should interpolate now that – apart from the loneliness and hard work involved in writing, or dealing with depressingly awful manuscripts – the circumstance common to us all seemed to be exposure to tung oil. This is used a lot industrially, in inks and varnishes for instance, and more particularly in liquid quick-drying erasers of type on manuscripts.' One of the writers suggested she consult his 'most helpful doctor', an electroacupuncturist in Auckland. This special-ist said she was suffering from too many antibiotics ('which I probably was') but suggested nothing else. He didn't detect any 2,4,5-T poisoning; she didn't then know she had been affected. He did, however, prescribe 'enormous quantities' of Nystatin tablets. 'To the best of my recollection he didn't say what they were for, and certainly nothing was said about the need to renew the prescription, or about diet. I imagined they were a kind of tonic. They were, of course, for candida albicans overgrowth, extremely common with this fatigue syndrome; I didn't learn this until long afterwards.'

Kate, with one book painfully finished and the other perforce handed to someone else to complete, departed with half a dozen jars of Nystatin tablets to meet commitments in Africa. Nystatin and the climate helped although walking was an ordeal and keeping to her long-planned schedule required constant effort. With difficulty she wrote two promised articles, but otherwise filled notebooks with material to write up in England, when, she thought, she surely would have left this baffling fatigue behind. In cold, damp England, with the Nystatin tablets finished, she became much worse.

'I simply couldn't believe what was happening to me. I had the joy of being with my children, I had exciting writing to do and all manner of excursions and parties were planned. All I wanted was to lie on a bed – and this behaviour in a person who normally travelled through life at 120 miles per hour, enjoying everything and everyone on the way.' She consulted a doctor who said she was over-tired, and suggested a holiday. 'I had to try to explain I *was* on holiday.'

As it happened she had booked, much earlier, to go on an archaeological cruise of the Mediterranean with a friend, so decided to go ahead. 'My poor long-suffering friend. She waited patiently while I dragged myself from one ruin to another. My memory was befuddled. I felt, when I was reading and making notes, that it was like trying to write on a sheet of glass; so few things made a real mark on my brain.' A few years later, when she was able to look at her friend's slides of the cruise, she could remember only half the archaeological sites shown. 'To see myself on the island of Rhodes, for instance, was an Alice in Wonderland experience. I couldn't remember having been transported there; I might have been Alice falling down a well.'

Kate returned from the cruise in a daze. 'I knew I must be ill, physically ill, but it was very hard to explain, even to my near and dear. It wasn't easy for them to adjust to a suddenly dopey, dozey, ultra-sensitive mother and mother-in-law. They must have thought, though didn't say, that I needed a psychiatrist.

'The next GP I went to wasn't so restrained. I see now that it was partly my fault. In a small community, where one is known, it's easy to say how one feels, and to be believed. But this was London and I was a stranger. I simply said to this doctor that I was tired, very very tired to the point where I couldn't do everyday ordinary things. And, because a friend had said that I might have Royal Free Disease (of which I hadn't previously heard), I mentioned this as a possibility. The doctor laughed in a peculiarly unpleasant way. I remember his words precisely. "Tired? Aren't we all tired! Show me someone who isn't. As for the so-called Royal Free Disease, that was proved to be nothing but hysteria." I didn't know enough to argue with him, and in any case didn't have the strength. He wrote me a prescription for valium, which I meekly accepted and later destroyed. And that was that. Or rather it was the beginning of my own researches. How dare he treat me like that? And how many other sufferers, perhaps less accustomed than I was to being assertive, were being reduced to quivering misery by doctors of his ilk?'

Her anger gave her enough energy to take herself to the British Medical Association library in Tavistock Square. With few clues, she searched through the catalogue, beginning with words such as 'fatigue' and 'Royal Free Disease'. Each medical paper gave references which led to others. She photocopied papers and found that a great deal of medical literature existed on the fatigue syndrome, with references from the first recognised outbreak, in Los Angeles in 1934.

Kate heard that a number of BBC staffers were ill with this disease which didn't seem to exist as far as GPs were concerned. One told her of being similarly derided by doctors but of feeling to some extent better after consultations with a naturopath. Kate also found some relief after fasting, following a mostly vegetable diet and taking capsules filled with dried herbs. Always optimistic, she thought perhaps she was better at last and accepted an invitation to India, as guests of Indians in the Jai Yogeshwar movement. Keeping one step ahead of exhaustion, she filled many notebooks with the intention of writing for publication when back in London. There extreme fatigue overcame her again. 'Fatigue and guilt make a wretched combination. Just as in Africa, so many people had shown me so much and, I felt, trusted me to write . . . and once again I couldn't.'

Tears came easily and her throat ached at any perceived unkindness or rebuke. Conversely she over-reacted to kindnesses. 'I learnt that this is called being "emotionally labile". Whatever it was, I had it. And my social life became problematic. At dinner with an agreeable man I fell asleep. When your head's down on the table next to the pepper steak, the situation isn't conducive to an interesting sequel.'

In London she then saw a doctor who knew her son and family. 'This pleasant man looked at me carefully while I was reciting my symptoms. I knew he was weighing a verdict of hysteria or anxiety-neurosis against the fact that there was no neurosis in my son's family. Suddenly a woman medical student, sitting in on the doctor's consultations as part of her training, spoke up excitedly. My symptoms, she said, were just like those of her own mother who had been forced to give up a lectureship in zoology because of inexplicable fatigue, depression and general weakness. The student and I began tossing symptoms and feelings back and forth, while the doctor followed first one, then the other of us, like a spectator at Wimbledon. Then he said with great conviction, "I've always said one should listen, really listen, to one's patients."

'I can't say how much it meant to have a doctor listen, and believe me. It didn't matter that he didn't have a name for the illness, let alone suggestions for treating it. He believed me.' Kate decided she must do more research.

She found the illness was given many different names in different countries, but there was no indication of possible cures. Then she became too weak to continue researching. One day someone told her of hearing a fragment of a radio talk about extreme fatigue. She phoned around until discovering that the BBC's Radio 4, in its medical programme, had run an item on M.E. or myalgic encephalomyelitis. It was an actual disease, and there was actually the M.E. Society of Great Britain, a support group for sufferers. 'Oh what a day that was! People who have never been ill with a derided and disallowed illness can have no idea how comforting it is to know you are not alone.'

The BBC programme had mentioned Professor James Mowbray of St Mary's Hospital medical school in Paddington. Kate tracked him down through miles of dingy corridors in the old Dickensian hospital where Alexander Fleming discovered penicillin. Professor Mowbray and his staff were friendly and welcoming. As a sideline to their main work they were giving injections of immunoglobulin to some M.E. sufferers. She was told that she should notice fairly soon if the injections were helping her. In her case they were not helpful, but, although each injection was painful, Kate returned several times because of the understanding shown her. 'It was quite a price to pay for a little human warmth.'

Then came the annual meeting of the support group, the Myalgic Encephalomyelitis Association of Great Britain. Kate met other

M.E. people, made notes, listened to doctors and, most importantly, to Dr Belinda Dawes, an M.E. sufferer herself, who devoted her practice to M.E. patients.

At her first consultation Kate learnt that Belinda Dawes had become ill just as she graduated from medical school in Adelaide, so ill that she had spent the next two years in bed at home or in hospital. The consultation was at the time of the Prince Andrew–Sarah Ferguson royal wedding, when many communities celebrated with parties. Dr Dawes showed Kate her heels, blistered from dancing at such a party until 4 a.m. 'I was amused and impressed. To have even half that energy would be wonderful.' Dr Dawes said she treated her patients' illnesses as she did her own.

The most important immediate treatment, Kate thinks, was being put on a diet containing no yeast in food or drink, and being prescribed quantities of Nystatin powder to take daily. In a matter of days this treatment for candida albicans overgrowth banished so much of her fatigue and depression that she thought she could perhaps write again, but this particular energy was not to return for a considerable time. She believes, from talking to many sufferers, that candidiasis nearly always accompanies the fatigue syndrome. Women are particularly prone to it but many men also benefit from a yeast-free regime, with Nystatin or Nilstat.

She had blood, sweat, urine and hair tests to check for mineral imbalances, and blood was taken for cytotoxic testing for food allergies. The laboratories concerned, Dr Dawes said, had a high level of accuracy. 'I protested that I didn't have food allergies; I'd already been to a conventional allergist in London who had found nothing. Dr Dawes just smiled.' These new tests showed varying deficiencies in a range of minerals, and extreme, moderate and slight sensitivities to many foods. Kate, put on an elimination and challenge diet, says she was still sceptical. 'These were foods I'd been eating all my life, and I'd had no symptoms such as migraine or pain – nothing. So I was excited and pleased at my reaction to an orange. I turned an orange-red and my skin prickled for about 20 minutes – all this after not having had my usual daily orange for a few weeks. I learnt later that this syndrome can produce all manner of unsuspected sensitivities. Or the hidden sensitivities may help produce the syndrome. I don't think anyone knows for sure, yet, how it happens. But happen it does.'

A regime of avoiding the foods she was most sensitive to, together with taking a prescribed list of minerals and vitamins, helped Kate's 'chop suey' brain. She could think more clearly and had a little more energy but was still far from her normal self. Dr Dawes then suggested she take a course of special injections known as EPD or Enzyme Potentiated Desensitisation. This would be expensive because of the cost of making the substance to be injected, more than 60 of the most common allergens in extremely tiny amounts, and potentiated or made more powerful by an enzyme extracted from a marine mollusc.

As all these previous treatments and tests had been expensive – 'the moment you walk into Harley Street you feel the money draining out of your purse' – and as Kate had no insurance and EPD was not covered by the National Health Service, she first sought out people who were already having EPD. All were enthusiastic, so she began the treatment. She carefully followed the instructions for immediately before and after each two-monthly injection, and enjoyed (after her restricted earlier diet) what Dr Dawes called 'eight on a plate' eating: small amounts of eight or so different foods at each meal, 'as if one were helping oneself from a smorgasbord'. This was to habituate herself to foods to which she had become sensitive. She could now eat oranges again, for instance, without reacting. Her one reaction was a moderately sore throat after each EPD treatment.

Meanwhile her physical and mental fatigue continued. 'I wasn't such a completely spineless jellyfish as I had been before beginning treatment from Dr Dawes, however. Then I'd felt just as I did one time when the accelerator cable on my car broke – I put my foot down on the accelerator, and nothing happened. For instance I'd decide to make a phone call or get up and get a drink of water – and nothing would happen. My muscles weren't doing what my brain told them to do. Most peculiar. Nasty, in fact, and it happened so often. To everyone else I looked normal enough, so how to explain I suddenly couldn't lift my foot to step on to a bus?'

Round this time Kate was talking to two fellow M.E. sufferers she had met at the society's annual meeting. They agreed they could tell one another things that non-M.E. people wouldn't understand. Kate said that quite often she'd thought how nice it would be to be dead, but –. The others interrupted, saying the trouble was her brain wasn't working well enough to figure out how, and in any case she'd have forgotten what she'd figured out before she had had time to put it into practice. 'That was exactly it. We laughed.

'I hope that doesn't sound flippant. The illness had made all three of us think about oblivion, release through suicide. But we were basically happy people, to whom the depression of M.E. seemed an overlay, something imposed on us, as it were. It was different with one of my friends, a university lecturer who killed himself after several years with M.E. He had never come to terms with a traumatised childhood, and the load of this illness became too heavy to bear. One night the depression peculiar to M.E. turned into a final despair.

'Hope and faith in eventual recovery and a fighting spirit can be, literally, vital for M.E. people.'

After her third EPD injection Kate was walking with her daughter in London when she said, imprudently, 'I've felt a twinge'. Her daughter was understandably alarmed. 'I explained it was a twinge of wellbeing, of happiness. It had been two years since I'd felt anything like that.' One twinge doesn't make a well person, but after her fourth EPD treatment Kate felt almost herself again. She returned to New Zealand and was active, physically and mentally, in an organisation she chaired, and began to pick up the pieces of her life. Writing, however, was still difficult. She had been told EPD was available in Australia but the promised arrangements fell through. As the months went by, Kate says, she felt as if she were 'an old torch battery, becoming dimmer by the day'. She became so fatigued again that she decided she must use her savings and return for treatment in London.

Time was limited so she arranged to have three more EPD treatments at six-weekly intervals instead of eight-weekly, as before. Dr Dawes was away when the second treatment was due so Kate arranged to have it from Dr Len McEwen. He had developed EPD in 1966 when he was a pharmacologist at St Mary's Hospital and medical school. It was originally only for hay fever sufferers but Dr McEwen gradually realised that his vaccines had the potential to desensitise people suffering from food and dust sensitivities.

'Dr McEwen talks to all his patients and he was running late – 8 p.m. He set up a television set in his waiting room so that those of us still waiting could watch, with him, a Thames TV programme on his own work. Patients and other doctors appeared on the programme, too. It was all most convincing, most cheering. Those of us still waiting for our EPD felt we were extremely fortunate.'

Dr McEwen told Kate that Belinda Dawes had worked on the nutritional and anti-candida aspects which he himself now used to complement EPD and stressed that he particularly wanted to teach more doctors. 'He said, "If I die tomorrow, I don't want the treatment to die with me." He explained that he has an immunologist making the vaccines in a laboratory attached to his own house at Henley-on-Thames, but that he hoped one of the big chemical companies would one day take over, and that the treatment would be available on the National Health Service. I fervently agreed. I'd met so many people who had really benefited, but many more who simply couldn't afford the treatment. Making the vaccine is so expensive.'

On her way from New Zealand to London this second time, and on her return journey, Kate addressed support groups in Los Angeles and talked to many people with the chronic fatigue and immune dysfunction syndrome. She found two main groups: those with CEBV or chronic Epstein-Barr virus, and those who are known as E.I. or environmentally ill. Those with CEBV had the same wide range of symptoms, and differences in the severity of the illness, as she had found among M.E. people in other countries. 'It was just that the diagnosed trigger-virus usually differed from country to country.'

Those who had become environmentally ill, the multi- or universal reactors, seemed in a worse situation even than those with the most severe post-viral syndrome. Some she had to speak to by phone as they had left the polluted air of Los Angeles for isolated mountain cabins, away from 20th-century chemicals.

'I met people whose case histories seemed so bizarre I shan't go into details. They definitely weren't neurotic. I can't stress that too much. They had an intelligent insight into their predicament and were struggling with enormous courage and ingenuity to get well again.' These people had become extremely sensitive to most foods and to virtually all chemical combinations devised in the past 40 years. The range extends from plastics, agricultural sprays, petrochemicals in general, synthetic fabrics, paper and inks to everyday purchases such as soap and toothpaste.

'In the States there are such extremes. I learnt of doctors more brutal to chronic fatigue sufferers than any I'd encountered elsewhere. Yet I also met some, and heard of many more, who seemed every sick person's dream of what a doctor could be. One flies from San Francisco to Los Angeles each month, for instance, and doesn't hesitate to consult with the environmentally ill outdoors if a completely 'safe' house isn't available. And of course anti-candida therapy was pioneered in the States by Drs Truss and Crook, and many others are involved in immune dysfunction research.'

The tone of many American newspaper and magazine articles nevertheless dismayed Kate, who found them negative, limited in their approach and inclined to feed medical scepticism about the reality of the illness. In the last months of 1987, for instance, she noticed headlines, in major publications, such as 'Mystery Illness Hitting Thousands of Yuppies – and There's No Cure!' And 'Fatigue "Virus" Has Experts More Baffled and Sceptical Than Ever'. Little seemed to be generally known about treatment and self-help, although a clinic giving EPD was operating in New York.

One problem, she thinks, is that wellknown Americans who have become ill with the fatigue and immune dysfunction syndrome are afraid to say so. This is particularly true of Hollywood where the illness is sufficiently prevalent to be known as 'the Hollywood Blahs'. Film director Blake Edwards (the *Pink Panther* series) let it be known he was a sufferer, but mostly there is fear of losing jobs or of not having contracts renewed, and a fear that CFS will be confused with AIDS. 'It's rather like the situation, years ago, when homosexuals were afraid to come out of the closet.' Kate points to a different climate of opinion in Britain, where the solo yachtswoman, Clare Francis, has let her illness be made public, and where the Dean of Westminster, the Very Reverend Michael Mayne, has written a book, *A Year Lost and Found*, about his experience, with the intention of helping other sufferers.

Kate says it is ironic that she had her own illness diagnosed and treated in Britain when in many respects her own country has more to offer, including EPD. 'I now have an excellent and knowledgeable GP. In every country, though, there are still only isolated pockets of medical knowledge and understanding. The usual pattern is, at best, mystification; at worst, derision and hostility.'

She discovered, on her return, that New Zealand is the leader in organised group support. The Australia-New Zealand Myalgic Encephalomyelitis Society (ANZMES), with regional support groups, was established in Auckland by M.E. sufferer Toni Jeffreys and her husband, Jim Brook-Church. They produce a periodical, *Meeting-Place*, which Kate describes as 'a cornucopia of facts, theories and exchange of ideas – by far the best publiction I've seen anywhere for chronic fatigue people, whatever triggered their illness.'

A recent questionnaire from ANZMES, she says, helped clarify her own experience.

The four symptoms which most distressed her were, in order of importance: mental fogginess, physical weakness and depression linked with candida albicans overgrowth. Her four biggest difficulties were inability to write, problems walking and keeping awake, scepticism and hostility from some doctors, and problems conveying her state to family, friends and work colleagues. The things she found most helpful were Nystatin, nutritional advice and food supplements, EPD, adopting a positive attitude while using visualisation and affirmations, and family warmth and support.

'If facts about M.E. and the chronic fatigue and immune dysfunction syndrome generally had been available to me and countless others when we first became ill, we would have had a far better chance of recovery, and not have lost so many years of our lives.' – CCC.

THERESA

Cycling, skiing and choral singing, as well as a demanding job, meant that Theresa, a Londoner in her 40s, had to keep 'supremely fit' and organise her life carefully so that she had time and energy for all her interests. For 10 years she had been superintendent of a small hospital for handicapped children, and had just returned from taking part in a French cycling club's 90-kilometre road rally when disaster struck.

'I would have said I was completely physically fit. I relished cycling six miles each way through London traffic to work, and had just organised a demonstration against juggernauts using the Embankment, so traffic would be easier for cyclists.

'But now I look back I realise I had a lot of turbulence in my life. I am actually an occupational therapist and it was this qualification which had given me my job, a combination of hospital matron, headmistress and administrator. But the new National Health people thought my position anomalous so had put another layer of administration on top of me. This wasn't easy to accept after 10 years. At the same time things were going a little wrong in a personal relationship – hardly surprising, considering the new strains of work relationships. But I felt I was coming to grips with the situation and accepting my changed role.

'This day in May 1984 I suddenly began to feel nauseated at work. I felt most peculiar. My knees and ankles hurt and my legs were constantly twitching. I couldn't possibly bike home but a colleague gave me a lift in a van. My dinner date had to be cancelled.'

Theresa went to work by bus the next day but had to go home early – 'the sort of thing that had never happened to me before'. An extremely severe headache almost blinded her. Then her joints became so painful that she spent the weekend in bed with her wrists, elbows and knees supported by cushions. A doctor consulted by phone said that she could have glandular fever, and suggested aspirin until she was well enough to go to the surgery for a test.

A week after becoming ill, Theresa 'tottered' back to work. She was surprised to find a colleague, who lived in the same area, also suffering from joint pains. (This woman, who led a sedentary life, recovered in about a month although the pain returned if she walked any distance.) Theresa told her GP about this other case, but he dismissed it. Glandular fever tests were negative, but as she was still in such pain her doctor suggested a short-lived sero-negative arthritis, and prescribed pain killers.

'In the next few days I was extremely ill. I would wake and feel just as if I had run 100 miles. I was too tired and achey to get out of bed to make a cup of tea. On one of these days I should have been on a cycle outing from London to Brighton. I lay in bed feeling I'd ridden the course several times over.When I had to go downstairs, I'd have to rest half-way up on my return as I could feel the power drain out of my leg muscles.'

Then came a time of partial remission although the joint pain continued. She returned to work, travelling by mini-cab or public transport. Some days she was particularly aware of the puzzling lack of power in her legs. If she did too much with her arms, they would run out of power too. Nearly two months after her first illness she felt well enough to accompany a group of handicapped children on a short holiday.

'I spent the first day with them at the beach, helping them to swim, swinging them about in the water, then later bathing, feeding and putting them to bed. We sat out for drinks and a meal on the terrace of a stately home we were staying in, then I played the grand piano for everyone. I had worked very hard to "prove" myself to the staff, because, as the superintendent, I didn't normally look after the children's daily needs.

'This day was probably the catalyst of my really severe illness. I woke the next morning so tired I didn't have energy to eat, and could cope only if I lay on the floor. I was taken home, chastened, to go straight to bed. I missed singing in a concert the next day, of course, and my GP gave me two weeks' sick leave, citing sero-negative arthritis. Again I had periods of complete exhaustion, then days when I felt a little better.' Her choir was to be the guest choir at the prestigious Aix-en-Provence music festival, and she was determined to go. Rehearsals were exhausting. She had to lean on a church pew for support while standing to sing. She went back to work, collapsed and was brought home. Her GP gave the impression that he thought she was imagining her symptoms. When she said to him, 'I've come about this illness,' his reply was, 'What illness?'

She says this made her 'very defensive and unhappy. Did he really think that somebody who had been so active would just give it all up and become a neurotic individual? My doctor gave me more time off work but dismissively filled in the certificate with the words, "pains down right arm". I'd told him my right wrist and elbow had been so painful I'd been unable to brush my teeth or do my hair properly, but I wasn't sure he believed me as there was no obvious muscle weakness.'

Hospital tests for arthritis were negative. Again Theresa felt the staff thought her symptoms were 'all in the mind'. She managed to take part in the music festival in France, although feeling she didn't sing well or very accurately. Then she heard of someone who had a similar illness. 'I felt so happy to talk to somebody who understood me. This woman had been ill for 18 months and didn't know what was the matter as all her tests had been negative. But I took her advice and went to a homoeopath.'

The homoeopath warned her that the remedy might give drastic results but that it would work. She spent the next three days frequently urinating, but since then has never experienced the same level of joint pain. She was able to sleep without her supporting pillows, and could sit down without first consciously arranging her limbs. No subsequent homoeopathic remedies were as successful.

Her life fell into a circumscribed pattern. Most days she could go to work, late, and come home early to flop on to settee or bed, too tired for any of her old activities although she managed to stay in the choir. Usually she was too tired to talk so lost contact with friends. 'My treats were small walks in a park, or being driven to a nice spot – although I was a bit querulous: "How far will we have to walk?" My house got grubbier but I was too exhausted to do any housework, and too exhausted to organise a cleaner. I put on weight – my body cried out for more food for more energy. When I had a good day it was surpising how much I could do in my garden. And a portable electronic typewriter helped as otherwise I'd be too tired to write more than a line. With my new typewriter at least I could manage a little more.

'What worried me extremely was my memory. I seemed to forget everything. I'd go to a meeting, agree to action, and then not remember what went on. I found it difficult to use words correctly, and my brain seemed to be made of cottonwool. I just could not think straight, and had no initiative. At least the staff at work could see I was ill – I would become a strange grey shade before a collapse. I also wept at the drop of a hat, and couldn't explain this as I didn't feel depressed. Sometimes tears would roll out of my eyes, or a minor upset such as a bus driver asking me to move along would set me off.'

Theresa saw a television programme on athletes and muscle exhaustion. An experiment suggested that bicarbonate of soda, taken before a run, had an effect on the lactic acid built up with exercise. She experimented herself with a teaspoonful and found it helped. Too much changes electrolyte balance so she didn't take bicarbonate of soda too often, but believes it has been a great help during the past two years.

Soon after this she learnt that she could take early retirement on grounds of ill health. She went to New Zealand for a long holiday and there, at last, she learnt what her illness was. A GP diagnosed M.E., put her on a yeast-free diet and prescribed Nystatin and multi-vitamins. Within six weeks she was a new person. 'I could feel a gradual improvement but one morning I woke up and felt as if I had my brain back. To have a clear head – what a marvellous feeling!'

Theresa was still not completely better, but being able to remember and to think clearly was a tremendous leap forward. Back in London she continued with the regime prescribed by the New Zealand doctor she had consulted. Creative visualisation, meditation and relaxation have played an important part in her progress, she says. For the past 18 months she has been using Reiki, or the Radiance Technique, an ancient Japanese healing technique to balance her body.

Her cycling is still limited to trips to nearby shops but she has had two gentle skiing holidays and finds that a weekly yoga class is strengthening her muscles. She has been having EPD at a homoeopathic hospital, and is sure it is helping her.

'Now, less than four years since this illness struck, I have made enough progress to be back playing my part in society. I work part-time at several enjoyable jobs, working at my own pace which I know is highly important. I have learnt not to take on too much, but I volunteered to run a large M.E. support group. Telephone calls from members needing support take up much of my time – on reflection I do probably work a 40-hour week.

'I am now certain I will regain all my old zest for life. I recognise that I may never cycle in a rally again, but M.E. has pointed me in other directions, for work and relaxation, so I whisper a cautious thankyou to this strange disorder, feeling sure that it need not always be with me.' – CCC

VIRUSES, AGENTS OF CHANGE

> We live in a dancing matrix of viruses; they
> dart, rather like bees, from organism to organ-
> ism, from plant to insect to mammal to me and
> back again and into the sea, tugging along
> pieces of this genome, strings of genes from
> that, transplanting grafts of DNA, passing
> around heredity as though at a great party.
> LEWIS THOMAS, *Lives of a Cell*, 1974.

The advent of AIDS, along with a global increase in viral illness, is
stimulating the revision of many ideas about the causes of disease.
Medical researchers are re-assessing old theories about the nature
of viral epidemics. Funds are being poured into prestigious insti-
tutes such as the U.S. National Cancer Institute, the Atlanta
Disease Control Center and the Pasteur Institute in Paris. The
resulting research is discovering many 'new' viruses, and the
realisation that weakened and mutated versions of the same virus
may produce differing symptoms. The health of future generations
will probably relate more to persistent viruses and the diseases
associated with them than to the relatively straightforward acute
viral infections.[1]

When the chronically unwell person complains about 'going
down with a virus', he or she is being touched by place and history,
by the health of generations before. The most mysterious and
misunderstood of disease agents, viruses are far more than they
seem to be. The word virus comes from the Latin for *slimy liquid,
stench, poison*. An appropriate derivation – for viruses rose out of the
primordial ooze to cohabit the globe along with the species that
followed after. The ultimate parasites, depending on their hosts,

they hide in the genes, passing down the generations and connecting us with all living things. Viruses are now seen as vehicles for the exchange of DNA between organisms and species, modifying, trimming and pruning every living species.[2]

Viruses have brought the scourges of smallpox, 'flu, yellow fever, Lassa fever, poliomyelitis, glandular fever and epidemic encephalitis; of chicken pox, measles, rubella, herpes, shingles and encephalitis lethargica. They are involved in warts, some cancers (particularly lymphomas), with up to 80 per cent of cervical cancers having a viral cause. They are now thought to be important in such disparate diseases as some types of depression, rheumatoid arthritis, multiple sclerosis and schizophrenia.

The Atlanta Center for Disease Control reported in 1986 that viruses which are already present in normal, healthy organisms become more virulent by repeated contact infections. These findings were confirmed that same year by the Soviets who reported that viral epidemics are particularly likely to build up in groups where young and old are combined. When the young, with their immature immune systems, have lowered immune competency, they can draw viral particles from their elders, incubate the virus within their own bodies, and reinfect their elders. Today's increasing virulence of viruses may be due, not to the viruses themselves, but to the increasing weakness of the organisms they inhabit. Healthy immune responses of many individuals are necessary to keep viral epidemics at bay.

Viruses consist simply of protein-coated molecules of the building blocks of life, either RNA or DNA. Both types are involved in chronic fatigue syndrome with RNA enteroviruses thought to be more significant. These include the Coxsackies, the poliovirus, and Echoviruses which flourish in the digestive tract. All the herpesviruses have been discovered in CFS patients, with a rapid increase since the early 1980s of the new human herpesvirus 6 (HHV6, formerly called the Human B cell lymphotropic virus).

Unable to reproduce themselves, viruses commandeer living cells to use their reproductive ability for their own reproduction. Thus healthy cells become virus factories, being weakened or killed in the process. The process is complex, but can be summarised in a simplified working model of what happens when a retrovirus invades a muscle cell[3] (see diagram adapted from M.E. Newsletter,

U.K., Autumn, 1987).

1.   The virus enters the bloodstream by any of a number of ways – through lesions, the respiratory tract, from bone marrow, the digestive system.

2.   In penetrating and commandeering a cell, the protein coat of the virus slips off, and its RNA viral gene is deposited on the invaded cell's RNA.

3.   Using the commandeered RNA, the activated genes make new virus cells, which escape from the cell, either killing it or weakening it in the process.

4.   RNA viral particles persist inside the cells, apparently blocking normal production of energy from the mitochondria by disrupting normal enzyme production and activity, and affecting mitochondrial structure.

5.   Enzyme deficits lead to lactic acid build-up when muscle cells are required to produce energy for movement.

British M.E. researcher Dr David Smith believes this working model explains the loss of energy, the cramps and muscle pains which often occur on exercise. 'The cure would obviously be to get rid of the virus sitting on the RNA. Therefore we would need an antiviral medication, to prevent the RNA entering new cells, or to promote the expulsion of this RNA inside the cell.'[4]

Viral Effects
Even supposedly 'mild' viruses such as those related to influenza can wreak a large number of previously unsuspected body changes. An Italian study (1980) under the direction of allergist Professor Lino Businco of Rome University listed the following pathological changes wrought in guinea pigs by chronic, recurring influenza: a vast impoverishment of lymph tissue – thus reducing the immune mechanism of the lymphatic organs; changes and lesions in the adrenal glands; loss of thyroid and renal function; hardening of parts of the lung; slight liver degeneration; severe degenerative

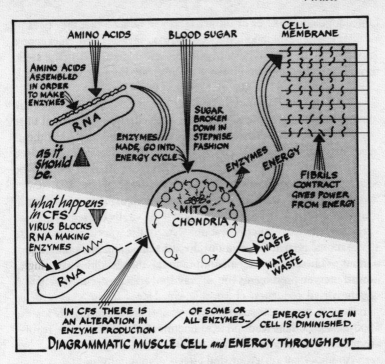

AMINO ACIDS   BLOOD SUGAR   CELL MEMBRANE

AMINO ACIDS ASSEMBLED IN ORDER TO MAKE ENZYMES

RNA

as it should be.

ENZYMES MADE, GO INTO ENERGY CYCLE

SUGAR BROKEN DOWN IN STEPWISE FASHION

ENZYMES   ENERGY

what happens in CFS
VIRUS BLOCKS RNA MAKING ENZYMES

MITO CHONDRIA

FIBRILS CONTRACT GIVES POWER FROM ENERGY

RNA

CO_2 WASTE

WATER WASTE

IN CFS THERE IS AN ALTERATION IN ENZYME PRODUCTION / OF SOME OR ALL ENZYMES— / ENERGY CYCLE IN CELL IS DIMINISHED.

DIAGRAMMATIC MUSCLE CELL and ENERGY THROUGHPUT

atrophy of the skin and hair bulbs; degenerative atrophy of the heart muscle. The authors conclude that persistent forms of influenza may, through the atrophy of the heart and degeneration of the adrenal and other endocrine glands, be 'at the root of the pathogenesis of asthenia' – debility, feebleness, thinness, lack of energy and drive and inability to handle physical and emotional stress.[5]

Persistent viruses and their causative role in allergies were first reported in 1977. A team headed by S. Ida found that viruses can cause the release of histamines and other factors from the gut and lungs with ensuing allergic reactions.[6]

Amelia Nathan Hill, founder of the British association Action Against Allergy, comments that members of her organisation reported viral infections preceding the development of their allergies. 'From a survey which Action Against Allergy carried out, we were able to establish that most allergics noticed that they first became allergic after some kind of infection, the most common being glandular fever or influenza. Some noticed that they became allergic after childhood illnesses such as measles and chickenpox. Many children are now born allergic, and a virus or bacteria could well explain how an illness like this can be passed on and is increasing at such a rate as allergy is today.'

Lack of energy, muscle fatigue and weakness are important aspects of the chronic fatigue syndrome. Various explanations are given. Most disturbances in energy metabolism involve enzyme pathway abnormalities. Specific enzyme deficiencies in purine metabolism have been suggested as being involved in the muscle symptoms associated with CFS (see previous diagram).

Abnormal electric impulses in muscles have been picked up in several M.E. studies and are thought to be virally caused.[7] Japanese researchers used 'microvibration' tests to discover 'invisible minute vibrations' related to 'emotions, hypothalamic and autonomic functions'. These tests revealed vibrational abnormalities correlating with nervous problems in depression and post-viral cases.[8] A generalised reduction or specific imbalances in the energy fields related to specific organs or body systems are major features in the physiological landscape in acupuncture and bio-energetic regulatory medicine.

An important review of viral effects of immunity and the nervous system was recently made at the Scripps Clinic and Research Foundation in California.[9] It should be required reading for all physicians dealing with CFS patients. Researchers Michael Oldstone MD and Peter Southern PhD, describe widespread changes to all types of cells, endocrine glands, T lymphocytes, enzyme functioning, and to the production of histamines and hormones (including insulin). In a paper in *The New England Journal of Medicine*, they outline the discovery that persistent viral infections can alter the physiological function of cells without destroying their own life-sustaining functions. Any sheepfarmer, putting his sheep through the counting gate, will appreciate this point, which raises many questions about cell-ratios and absolute numbers. Both farmers and researchers are more likely to count numbers, rather than make evaluations of the individual health status of sheep or cells.

Discussing the medical consequences of persistent viral infections, Oldstone and Southern say: 'Destruction of relatively few cells that are required for specialised functions, such as neurotransmission, hormone production and secretion, immune responses, or myocardial contraction, can be disabling or even life threatening.' They also make the point that the immune status of the host is crucial to the extent of pathological changes.

A growing number of neurologists and virologists are now resurrecting the hypothesis that chronic viral infections are symptomatic of systems that are breaking down, and that those with healthy defence mechanisms can carry dormant, non-infective viruses in their bodies. This concept was aired by Wilhelm Reich, the Viennese-emigré psychoanalyst and medical researcher, who was imprisoned in the United States for persisting with unorthodox medical treatments aimed at reinforcing body energies. Such treatments are now widely used by alternative practitioners, and are under serious examination in research centres in the United Kingdom, the United States and Japan.

'In his later years Reich was interested in cancer and the breakdown of organisms over time. He identified small fragments of breakdown particles which were endogenous to the organism. These were fragments of things that were actually being generated by the organism. They weren't coming from outside. I feel that maybe that's what's happening in a lot of these illnesses – viral diseases and so on,' AIDS clinician Steven Thiry MD, says. He is directing a clinical research project aimed at boosting levels of electromagnetic energies in severely ill volunteers at Mt Zion Hospital in San Francisco.[10]

Thiry explains that what we identify as viruses may actually be the breakdown of formerly healthy, functioning tissue. 'There is also infectivity – these particles have life properties that can be transmitted to other organisms.'

The immune similarities between AIDS and CFS are outlined in the next chapter. Laboratory tests show many similar pathogens and immune changes. Both have persistent bacteria, persistent parasites, and many persistent viruses in common. One difference may be the extent of the enzyme damage. An Australian study showed that AIDS patients have an average 30 per cent of normal levels of adenosine deaminase and four enzymes involved in nucleic acid metabolism.[11] No studies on CFS have had similar results.

Those with persistent herpesviruses may face more difficulties.

These can include inflammation of the heart, brain and lungs, chronic hepatitis, bleeding sores,marked decreases in both red and white blood cells, and brain lesions in addition to the central nervous symptoms generally found in CFS. Herpesviruses may predominate in the 25 per cent of severely ill patients whose illness simply goes on and on. They live like grey shadows of themselves – sleeping badly, mostly severely depressed, incapacitated from time to time, sometimes a little better, but only rarely feeling anything like well.

'A Unifying Virus' for CFS

Many different viruses have been involved in the chronic fatigue syndrome under its many names. The principal ones include the five herpesviruses: Herpes simplex viruses 1 and 2, varicella-zoster virus, Epstein-Barr virus, cytomegalovirus; the enteroviruses: Echo ('flu) viruses, poliovirus, and the Coxsackies; arboviruses (related to insects); rubella, vaccinia (a cattle virus), hepatitis A and B, measles.

The more viruses are discovered, the more confused the picture becomes. Many are similar to the viruses found in AIDS, yet, as we know, the disease process is not fatal, and quite different. A worldwide network of medical researchers who are interested in the mystery epidemics that have occurred this century continue to seek answers. Among this group are Dr Melvin Ramsay, the British champion of M.E.; Dr J. G. Parish, another British doctor who has made wide-ranging studies into the background of M.E.; and Lawrence Kelly, an Ann Arbor, Michigan, virologist.

Encephalitis lethargica caused a serious European encephalitis epidemic (as distinct from the Spanish 'flu) from 1915-1928. The neurologist Oliver Sachs painted a chilling portrait of its effects in his book, *Awakenings*.[12]

Ex-lethargica sufferers featured prominently in a European and British crime-wave in the 1920s. There was concern even then that these ex-servicemen had become criminal through no fault of their own, and that society had the moral obligation to cure them rather than incarcerate them.

The Matheson Commission was set up in the United States to investigate the encephalitis epidemics. Its final report in 1929 traced the origin of the lethargica virus back to the trenches of World War I. It explained the virulence of the early lethargica encephalitis outbreaks as arising from the conditions suffered by the troops. 'A "cradle" for the virus in the war-time conditions of malnutrition, stress, weather exposure, exhaustion – a cradle which, in first promoting outbreaks in ill-fed, rain-soaked, constantly bombarded trench troops, triggered the carriers, and through the multiple passage in youthful, virus-free conscripts, adjusted the virus to its human hosts.'[13]

Although there is some dissension, HHV6, offspring of lethargica, appears to be a recombitant virus since antibodies to all the other human herpesviruses fail to recognise it. It is now believed to be related to avian herpesviruses, such as the well-studied Marek's chicken virus. Dr Paul Cheney, the Lake Tahoe doctor who drew world attention to chronic Epstein-Barr virus, is one who accepts this theory. He believes that HHV6 is a new virus, and that a lot can be learnt about it by looking at what Marek's chicken virus does to chickens.

'Small chicks and old chicks do not get this disease as much as middle-aged chicks,' he told a Lake Tahoe audience.[14] 'Female chickens are much more likely to become ill than male chickens. And stress plays a role too. They've actually studied this. How do you stress a chicken? Vaccinate it, de-beak it, fire off loud noises. They've been able to increase the expression of the disease in chickens by stressing them. I think many of you who may have this disease are aware of what stress factors can do to your disease.'

HHV6 is moving fast through the world's population. It has been found in both blood and saliva. Its incidence in the United States has jumped from 2 per cent of the general population to 30 per cent in just four years. Researchers expect it to reach the same prevalency as EBV in the next few years, about 90 per cent of the population. At present, only 5 per cent of those showing evidence of infection with HHV6 appear to have a chronic illness attributable to it. Only about 20 per cent of those have recovered completely. So far most victims have been aged 25-45, with the majority in their 30s. Cheney believes the eventual incidence of people who are ill with HHV6 (as distinct from the healthy carriers) will be about 12 million in the United States, and that the virus will have no boundaries.

'The very existence of CEBV support groups – rising out of practically nothing to over 200 now in a very few years – is one

factor,' he told Hillary Johnson of *Rolling Stone* magazine in 1987.[15]
'Secondly, an epidemic occurring among 40-year-olds. You would
no more expect an epidemic in 40-year-olds with a herpesvirus, if it
were an ancient virus, than you would expect an epidemic among
40-year-olds of chicken pox. Thirdly, if this were an old disease,
how could we possibly have missed it for all these years? There are a
large number of patients who are subtle and may not be that sick,
but there are patients who are really quite incredible and I just can't
believe the medical profession could have watched this – missed
this – for decades, or millenia.'

SELECTIVE TARGETS

Viruses target different organs, and even different cells. HIV, the
AIDS virus, targets the T cells; the herpesviruses, such as EBV, the
B cells. Herpesviruses are latent in almost everyone. Once infected
by EBV during glandular fever or 'mono', B cells proliferate and
become 'immortalised', as scientists put it. The immortalised cells
are destroyed by killer T cells in a battle that makes the patient feel
extremely ill. The threat is never wholly eliminated, however. A few
B cells harbour the virus (about one in a million) in otherwise
healthy individuals. There is a kind of armed truce, with the T cells
keeping them under control.

If latent herpesviruses are present (as they are in 90 per cent of
people), the CFS-type immune damage is conducive to uprisings of
virally infected B cells. The immune brigades are called out and
civil war will rage. As long as neither side wins, the patient will
experience all the symptoms of CFS. If the immune system wins,
the patient will return to full health. If the virus wins, however,
there will be serious physical and mental deterioration.

Human herpesvirus 6 (HHV6) goes further. It targets and
destroys B cells and therefore the source of antibodies. Like the
AIDS virus, HHV6 is a lytic virus which multiplies hundreds, even
thousands of times within each cell. As the cell bursts and dies, it
releases viral cells into the bloodstream. Not unsurprisingly, HHV6
upsets the balance of power between the immune system and any
latent viruses or other invaders.

It was originally thought that people with allergies would not
develop cancer. It is now known that cancers are associated not only
with the AIDS virus, but with the Epstein-Barr virus, hepatitis B,

cytomegalovirus and some other persistent viruses. A prolonged viral presence in the body and the accompanying overload on the immune system eventually impairs the body's ability to check malignant cells.

Such a scenario may sound like doom for that part of the human race confident of escaping AIDS. Yet, as has been noted earlier, HHV6 is also found in the bodies of perfectly healthy people, people unaware of any health problems whatsoever. The difference between those who are healthy, or 'always off-colour' or who are seriously ill with CFS increasingly looks like one of degree of immune strength or weakness.

Chapter 4   VIRUSES

1   Southern, P., and Oldstone, M.B.A., 'Medical Consequences of Persistent Viral Infection', Beth Israel Hospital Seminar in Medicine, *NEJM*, 314:6 359-67, 9.

2   Davis, B.D., 'Frontiers of the Biological Sciences', *Science*, 209:88, 1980.

3   Smith, David, 'A working model of the explanation of muscular fatigue in post viral syndrome', Myalgic Encephalomyelitis Association (U.K.) *Newsletter*, Autum 1987, p.4.

4   ibid.

5   Businco, L. et al., in *Clinica Europea*, Anno XIX, N5, September/October 1980.

6   Ida, S., Hooks, J.J. et al., 'Enhancement of IgE-mediated histamine release from human basophils by viruses; role of interferon', *J. Exp Med* 1977; 145; 892-906.

7   Jamal, G.A. & Hansen, S., 'Electrophysiological studies in the post-viral fatigue syndrome', *Jnl Neurology, Neurosurgery and Psychiatry* 1985; 48:691-4.

8   Nakagawa, T., Kawano, T. et al., 'A clinical and psychophysiological study of depression in internal medicine', *Psychosomatics*, 1976, 17:173-9.

9   Southern, P., and Oldstone, M.B.A., op, cit.

10   Interview with author.

11   'Enzyme test monitors AIDS progress', in *Australian Doctor*, 18 April 1986. Also personal correspondence with Dr Dick Chalmers, who headed the Mater Hospital research group, Brisbane.

12   Sachs, Oliver, *Awakenings*.

13   Report of a survey of the Matheson Commission, *Epidemic encephalitis; etiology, epidemiology, treatment*, New York; Columbia Univ Press, 1929; 179-81.

14   Johnson, H., 'Journey into Fear: The Growing Nighmare of Epstein-Barr Virus', *Rolling Stone*, 30 July and 13 August 1987.

15   ibid.

THE IMMUNE NETWORK

> As a net is made up by a series of ties, so everything in this world is connected by a series of ties. If anyone thinks that the mesh of a net is an independent, isolated thing, he is mistaken ... each mesh has its place and responsibilities in relation to other meshes.
>
> BUDDHA, 600 BC.

The rise of immune dysfunction syndromes and diseases is focussing the world's attention on the secret processes of the immune system. Speaking in New Zealand in 1988, Dr William Crook, author of *The Yeast Connection*, said: 'We know so little about the immune system. We are probably at the stage of understanding it as the world was of New Zealand when Captain Cook first mapped it.'

The immune system is the body's defence against every potential damaging factor in the environment. Intricate, intelligent, cooperative, combative, it is a networking organisation of red and white blood cells, antibodies and other protein substances, chemical messengers, hormones, bacteria and natural chemicals, enzymes, mitochondria, the lymphatic tissues, the thymus, spleen, brain and other glands.

Invading micro-organisms, viruses, air, food and abnormal body cells – all of these are processed, one way or another, by elements of the immune system. Its health is based on the health of the endocrine glands, and particularly the liver, spleen and thymus. The latter, where helper, killer and suppressor T cells are matured, is the overall director of the immune 'orchestra'.

The healthy immune system can defeat many viruses and bacteria and other infections, even body parasites. Cholera bacteria when taken into the body, for example, do not always cause cholera. The same was true with smallpox. Parasites and bacteria such as giardia lamblia, staphylococcus aureus (the H-bug), salmonella and campylobacter are life-threatening only to those with weakened immune systems. The herpesviruses are carried by 90 percent of the population, yet most are totally unaware of their presence. The AIDS virus is endemic in certain perfectly healthy South American and African tribes, and American AIDS specialists report that immunity is developing in some previously ill men.[1] There is no reason to doubt that a healthy immune system can also cope with the complex mix of viruses, bacteria and toxins that cause CFS.

THE IMMUNE ARMY

Major components of the immune system are grouped as follows:

NON-SPECIFIC IMMUNITY . . . one cell, many pathogens, immediate reaction

---

NATURAL KILLER CELLS recognise and destroy invaders on sight. They destroy tumours and virally infected cells by producing a cytotoxin, or cell poison.
NEUTROPHILS (or granulocytes) digest fungi, bacteria and debris.

SPECIFIC IMMUNITY . . . one specific cell, one specific pathogen . . . delayed reaction

---

Cell-Mediated Immunity

T CELLS patrol the body, destroying abnormal cells before they proliferate. A major part of cell-mediated immunity, they help regulate immune activity. There are different types of T cells.

HELPER CELLS enhance aggressive action against invaders.

SUPPRESSOR T CELLS cool the action down.

KILLER T CELLS recognise and destroy cancerous and virus-infected cells, after a previous encounter with them.

PHAGOCYTES AND MACROPHAGES are scavengers which engulf or devour fungi, bacteria and remove debris. They also signal the presence of invaders and can be called to battle by the T cells.

LEUKOTRIENES are chemical compounds that occur naturally in white blood cells. They are able to produce allergic reactions.

LYMPHOKINES are chemical signals and healing factors produced by T cells. They include interleukins 1-8; interferon, alpha, beta and gamma (stimulate immune cells and slow down viral replication); growth factors. All are integral in the immune response.

Humoral Immunity

B CELLS play a major part, staying close to the lymph nodes, producing antibodies against specific antigens. The blood then carries antibodies to the battle area.

ANTIBODIES (immunoglobulins): sticky protein particles that bind to bacteria, viruses and toxins or bring in phagocytes to devour invaders.

COMPLEMENT proteins lock on to pathogens and dissolve them.

The Immune Response

The following is a simplified outline of how the immune system responds to attack (see diagram on p.53). The first line of defence is given by cells called neutrophils (or granulocytes) and the natural killer cells. Complement proteins identify invaders for attack by the main army of phagocytes, macrophages and helper T cells. Communication is provided by chemical messengers (e.g. lymphokines), mainly emanating from helper cells.

Enzymes from the circulating complement system further disable invaders. B cells and the antibodies they produce (immunoglobulins, IgA, IgE, etc) then move into action. Antibodies, assisted by helper T cells and red blood cells, disable invaders. Suppressor T cells then deactivate helper T cells and B cells, and switch off the attack process.

Factors (other than viral) which weaken immune competency are fungal overgrowth,[2] which can lead to the development of autoimmune disease;[3] trace element deficiencies and heavy metals (such as lead, mercury and cadmium) in the body[4] which particularly affect enzyme and hormone functioning; excessive fatigue and continual exposure to infections. Continual infections may result in 'antigen overload', weakening and slowing down the immune response. All endocrine glands are susceptible to candida infestation, while the thymus and lymph glands are particularly sensitive to stress of any kind. Thus the stress factor is a crucial element in overall immune health, and particularly in CFS, because stress activates latent herpesviruses and upsets the body's natural balances.

Yet these same factors have differing effects on differing people. Understanding why and how this is so provides a sound platform for corrective measures. There is a growing suspicion that the highly processed nature of Western diet, with accompanying loss of vitamins and trace elements, may not provide the immune system with necessary nutrients.

In his introduction to *Food Allergy and Intolerances* (editor: Dr Jonathan Brostoff), the eminent physiologist and World Health Organisation consultant, Dr Morrell Draper, castigates modern diets and food technology, saying: 'It is obvious that nutritional science has at present no satisfactory understanding of what should constitute an adequate diet.' He supports the basic premise of the orthomolecular nutritionists, saying: 'Diet must provide, in addition to the molecules needed for vital functions, maintenance and energy, a further and variable supply of key molecules for the "non-nutritive" functioning of the defence system of the body.'[5]

THE IMMUNE ARMY IN ACTION.

 1. Invader multiplies

 2. Neutrophils and natural killer cells scavenge and destroy.

 3. Complement system proteins tag invaders.

 4. Macrophages scavenge and alert T helper cells.

5. T helper cells activate defence army.

 6. B cells produce antibodies against specific invaders (antigens)

 7. Antibodies disable specific invaders; further activation of complement system.

 8. Killer T cells destroy virus-infected and cancer cells.

 9. Suppressor T cells stop or slow the immune response and deter the body from attacking itself.

10. Some T and B cells are primed for instant defence if the same invader attacks again.

THE CFS IMMUNE RESPONSE

AIDS has educated the world as to the significance of tiny abnormalities in helper T cell and suppressor T cell ratios. The type of immune response found in early AIDS, the AIDS-related-condition, ARC, in allergies,and in early CFS is one of over-reaction, unlike the flattened response in cancer. Because suppressor T cells are reduced in number or are under-active, they fail to switch off T helper cells when they have done their job. The whole immune response continues for longer or with more vigour than it should. The body itself may be attacked. Malfunctioning suppressor cells also cause immune hyperactivity in illnesses such as rheumatoid arthritis, lupus and multiple sclerosis.

The British organisation Action Against Allergy's awards for Allergist of the Year (non-medical) for both 1986 and 1987 were given to the Surrey medical researcher and therapist, Tuula Tuormaa. In her 1987 prize-winning paper on the immune system, she describes similarities among the above diseases. 'They share defective T helper/T suppressor cell ratios, intracellular acidosis and hypoglycaemic episodes. All these are frequently combined with virus infections and/or food and chemical allergies,' she says.[6]

Normally there should be at least two helper T cells for every suppressor cell. In acute cases and in the early stages of CFS, the total number of both helper and suppressor cells is significantly reduced. In the chronic, longterm cases the helper cells are reduced until there is a near-inversion of the helper/suppressor ratio.[7] The number of suppressor cells keeps on growing until they turn off healthy helper cells. The result is a creeping deterioration in cell-mediated immunity.

The role of red blood cells in handling and inactivating potentially dangerous antigens may have been underestimated. Formerly viewed simply as carriers of oxygen, red cells are now known to be involved in allergic reactions and play a vital part in immune response. 'Though each individual cell has only a limited capacity to inactivate potentially dangerous antigens, antigen-antibody reactions are far more likely to be activated by red cells rather than white cells because of the overwhelming majority of the former,' Tuormaa says.[8]

Unique abnormalities in red blood cells in the blood of people with CFS are now being found. Dr Les Simpson, senior research

pathologist at the University of Otago in 1985 found stiffness and
deformities in blood cells from New Zealand's Tapanui 'flu victims.
This abnormality results in 'sticky blood', slower circulation and
poor delivery of oxygen and other nutrients of especial importance
to the brain.[9] The Australian edition of *Time*, 21 September 1987,
reported that Australian researchers 'nearly fell off their chairs'
when they found similarly deformed blood cells in 90 per cent of
CFS blood samples. 'We do a tremendous amount of blood and
tissue analysis here. Neither of us had seen anything like this,'
tissue pathologist Dr Tapen Mukherjee was reported as saying.[10]

A previously unsuspected effect of persistent viruses is a deple-
tion of neutrophils, part of the body's initial defence. These
neutralise the by-products of allergic and hypersensitive reactions
and prevent fungi from building up and causing systemic infection.
Digesting bacteria and debris, they literally 'clean up' the blood.
Neutropenia (low neutrophil levels) is found in CFS, AIDS and
ARC.

A basic aspect of the immune response is the antibody/antigen
reaction. Antibodies circulate throughout the body as sticky protein
particles of which there are five main types: IgA, IgD, IgE, IgM and
IgG. Each type of antigen has its own special function related to
particular types of circulating foreign invaders. None function
against pathogens hidden within cells. They bind to viruses, but
they do not kill them. That task is left to the natural killer (NK) cells
and the killer T cells. Any antibody deficiency will result in immune
deficiency; any excess can cause hypersensitivity. Abnormal levels
of antibodies are commonly reported in CFS as, for instance,
'IgA-lowered; IgM-raised'.

The woes of the body's defences continue. Evidence of the
fundamental weakening of the quality of the immune troops
surfaced in 1988 in British studies being carried out by Dr David
Smith and Professor Timothy Peters. Admittedly, their study
covered only 15 people with CFS, but all 15 had exactly the same
abnormality. This was a 20 per cent diminution of RNA (ribonucleic acid) within cells tested through muscle biopsies.

Dr Smith, a medical adviser to the U.K. M.E. Association,
commented in its Summer 1988 newsletter: 'In each of these cases,
despite the fact that the way in which they developed their Post Viral
Syndrome was different, and despite the fact that the virology being

looked at was also different, the common end finding was that they each had the same type of abnormality in their muscle.

'Most of this RNA is found inside a thing called a ribosome, which is really the engine of the muscle cell. Other parts of RNA have different functions, but it really can be looked upon as being part of the machinery that develops the power.'[11]

This finding is relevant to the muscle fatigue and weakness so common in CFS, no matter its background. For the effects of viruses on muscle cell RNA, see p.41.

Perhaps the most serious weakening of the immune troops in CFS is the dramatic reduction in numbers of natural killer (NK) cells in patients where the human herpesvirus 6 (HHV6) is present. Dr Cheney, Dr Daniel Peterson, Dr Anthony Komaroff and Dr Michael Caliguri found substantial NK reductions in more than half the Lake Tahoe patients tested. There was 0 per cent reduction in the healthy controls. NK cells, commandos of the immune system, are on constant patrol for invaders or unhealthy tissue. A crucial defence against cancer cells, they are thought to be the most important means the body has of containing latent herpesvirus infections.[12] Anthony Komaroff suggests that just as the symptoms of CFS are known to wax and wane, the health of the natural killer cells might ebb and flow as well.

A 1986 study on the cell-mediated immunity of New Zealanders with M.E.[13] revealed severe depression of cell mediated immunity in both those with M.E. and the supposedly healthy controls. (Cell-mediated immunity is one of the most important resistance factors to viral disease.)

The study was based on a similar one, comparing Australian homosexual and heterosexual males. The New Zealand study suggested that Australian homosexual men had immunity superior to the New Zealand controls. 'By international standards, our supposedly healthy controls look as though they have an immune problem,' team member Professor Campbell Murdoch of Otago Medical School, said. 'We are always told we are a relatively healthy people living in splendid isolation from the rest of the world. There is absolutely no illness for which New Zealand has the lowest rate in the world; for most of them we are among the highest.'

Regarding specific abnormalities, Professor Murdoch noted the presence of autoantibodies. 'Smooth muscle autoantibodies are the most common, as Dr Peter Behan has shown in Glasgow. These are particularly associated with liver dysfunction and chronic active hepatitis. They are in the blood vessels and in the tissues. Half the patients have a high immunoglobulin M which indicates an immune problem. Many develop low levels of iron, indicating that their iron metabolism is not functioning properly.'

Remarkable preliminary findings by Dr Peter Behan of Glasgow's Institute of Neurological Sciences were reported in the first issue of *InterAction*, the journal of the M.E. Action Campaign in Britain. Appearing in November 1988, the report showed that:

● Although B cells appear normal, they lack a particular antigen (a substance which stimulates the production of antibodies). This abnormality appears to be unique to M.E.

● When measuring the levels of Interleukin-1 Beta (a chemical messenger of the immune system) in M.E. sufferers, and comparing these with matched controls of normal people as well as with sufferers of certain other diseases, it was found that the average level in the normal control group was 20 titograms per millilitre. In people with rheumatoid arthritis the level was up to 51. In many people with M.E. the level was up to 20,000 ('This is not a typographical error,' says *InterAction*.)

So abnormal and so unexpected were the levels of Interleukin-1 Beta in the blood of M.E. sufferers that the laboratory doing the measurements thought there had been a mistake, and that pure Interleukin-1 Beta had somehow been added to the blood samples.

InterAction notes that Interleukin-1 Beta is known to

● turn on the production of other chemical messengers
● trigger fever
● act on the liver to displace protein production
● affect sugar metabolism
● break down cartilage and increase breakdown of muscle
● act on the nerve and muscle cells
● cause sleepiness and loss of appetite
● decrease white cell count

'The known effects of Interleukin-1 Beta could account for many M.E. Symptoms, especially the muscle, nerve and sleep phenomena,' *InterAction* comments. 'But perhaps the most interesting fact is that liver protein production and sugar metabolism are directly affected by this Interleukin. Imbalances in the liver and sugar metabolism are known to induce mood-swings and depression. Thus, for the first time, we could have an explanation for the high incidence of organic depression.'

As *InterAction* further points out, the cause of these abnormalities is not yet known. Nevertheless the importance of Dr Behan's most recent research findings must be obvious even to the most sceptical.

'FREE RADICALS' AND ANTI-OXIDANTS
Oxygen is regarded as essential to tissue and cell health, yet it can take toxic forms which combine with other chemicals to form destructive agents. These free radicals cause physiological changes to tissues and cells, just as oxidation can cause metal to rust.

There is increasing evidence that these free radical oxidative processes are the key to many disease processes – even to cot deaths.

The production of free radicals is encouraged by poor nutrition and diets that lack anti-oxidants – vitamins A, C and E, beta-carotene, the essential fatty acids, various amino acids and selenium. Low anti-oxidant protection weakens the lipid molecules in cell membranes.

Free radicals, oxidative processes and nutritional causes and corrective approaches are being widely studied throughout the world.

CORRECTING 'THE MILIEU'
Conventional immunologists and Western medicine in general are inclined to focus on the active agents of the body's defence system, such as T cells and B cells, when explaining the immune system. The nutritional, chemical and electromagnetic status of the body's cells and 'the milieu' – the intra-cellular and extra-cellular fluids and their environment – are central to the 'new' medicine.

The role of low density lipids and of amino acids and their cofactors (vitamins and minerals) in nourishing cells and metabolic pathways is a rapidly growing area of research and clinical application. Amino acids and lipids are the building blocks for the protein (bone, tissue and membrane) that makes up 75 per cent of the solid matter in the body. An adequate intake of all these elements is required for overall health and vitality, and immune functioning. The immune cells themselves are made from amino acids, and are formed with the help of vitamins, particularly C and the B complex, and trace elements.

Thus correction of 'the milieu' is the basis for many of the new therapies which are being picked up by some far-seeing doctors. They are moving into the chemically oriented approaches of physicians such as Dr Robert Erdman of Tunbridge Wells, UK, and Emanuel Revici, MD, the Rumanian-born New York-based specialist in immune disorders. Dr Revici's followers, whether they be qualified doctors or nutritional therapists, believe him to be a principal medical thinker of this century.

Dr Revici was celebrated for his successful treatment of cancer and chronic pain and disease more than 40 years ago. The Revici view of nature is one of biological dualism – the balance of opposing forces: electrostatic v electromagnetic, positive charge v negative charge, anabolic v catabolic; acidosis v alkalosis; sodium v potassium; and so on. His theories and the success of his approach provide a whole new horizon to the body's defence system and illustrate the complex processes in the type of physiological breakdown presented by persistent viruses, allergies and immune dysfunction.

Tom O'Connor of San Francisco, author of *Living With AIDS: Reaching Out*, is one who vouches for the success of the Revici method. Lynn Anderson MD, of Butte Falls, Oregon, one of several United States doctors using Revici's therapies, finds it is tailored to the correction of immune dysfunction. 'His outstanding contribution is the documentation of the defence mechanism far beyond the immune system alone, in particular, the elaboration of the lipid defence mechanism.' Anderson says that unlike modern medicine, which is basically limited to biochemistry, Dr Revici draws heavily on physical chemistry. It is impossible to understand his approach without studying his major treatise, *Research in physiopathology as basis of guided chemotherapy*.[14]

Applying Dr Revici's theories to CFS creates a new dimension to the illness, in that CFS involves a failure in the lipid defence. Treatment with diet and specially developed lipids involves balancing the body in a number of ways.

Lynn Anderson says: 'If the analysis shows the patient is anabolic you would give anti-anabolic or catabolic treatment. And vice versa if the patient is catabolic.' The opposing catabolic/anabolic forces

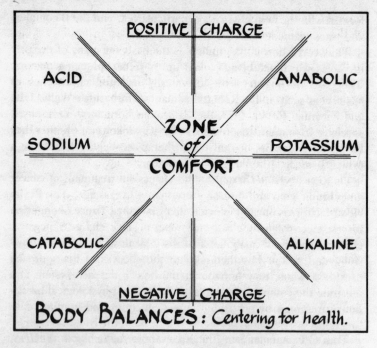

POSITIVE | CHARGE

ACID   ANABOLIC

ZONE
of
SODIUM   POTASSIUM
COMFORT

CATABOLIC   ALKALINE

NEGATIVE | CHARGE

BODY BALANCES: Centering for health.

relate to the processes of reconstruction (anabolic) and of destruction (catabolic). Every day the body goes through a complete catabolic/anabolic cycle, and both phases are indispensable to wellbeing.

Anderson finds that CFS patients with more acute symptoms such as anxiety and depression, musculoskeletal pain, severe and frequent reactions to foods and environmental factors, sleep disturbances and burning on urination, are over-catabolic. Patients who are more simply fatigued – 'often profoundly fatigued' – are over-anabolic.

Paradoxically, the catabolic patients often show immediate and even dramatic responses to anabolic treatments or alkalinising agents whereas the anabolic patients take a very long time to respond. Emphasising the effects of chemical residues in the latter patients, Anderson says that aggressive and longterm detoxification programmes are often needed.[15]

Explaining the role of lipids in the immune system, Dr Revici says:[16] 'The body's defences react against an antigen through several specific phases. The first phase concerns the breaking down of the complex antigen through the action of hydrolic enzymes manufactured by the neutrophilic granulocytes in a process similar to that of digestion. This is followed by a lipidic phase followed in turn by a phase corresponding to coagulant antibodies, such as agglutin and precipitin. This phase is followed by a fourth and final one mediated through globulinic antibodies (humoral immunity).'

The lipid level is the one at which Dr Revici bases his anti-viral treatment. He uses specially prepared forms of fatty and amino acids to support the body's lipidic defences including cell membranes, to correct pH levels and to counteract catabolic or anabolic imbalances. One of the most serious consequences of an anabolic imbalance is the heightened activity of bacteria, viruses, fungi and parasites in an alkaline environment.

A report on his work[17] says: 'According to Revici, defensive reactions occur because the body is organised in a hierarchy of levels, each level being an environment to the next lower level . . . a cell has to maintain and defend the function of its lower levels . . . Similarly the tissues maintain the cells through the interstitial fluids, the organs maintain the tissues through the lymphatic fluids, and the organism maintains the organs through the blood. When an alkaline imbalance on the cellular level becomes severe, the tissues will adjust (defend) with acidity, as if trying to force acid into the overly alkaline cells. If this also becomes too severe, the organs will adjust with alkalinity, in an attempt to mediate the acidic tissues.

'Therapeutically, you need to support the underlying imbalance, so that the higher level gives up its defence, and then you treat the next lower level. Just as you might peel off the layers of an onion, ultimately you can get back to the original imbalance. Although the total picture may be complicated, the level manifesting is the only one that needs immediate attention.'

Dr Revici has created an extraordinarily complex physiological scenario. No wonder that most medical professionals and the pharmaceutical industry are not excited. Yet the simple answers to the chronic fatigue syndrome presented as fact by many top medical researchers are a sore point with sufferers and specialist doctors. They feel there is far more to what is going on than can be explained by this virus or that lymphocyte. Campbell Murdoch feels that many virologists are way off beam, since the business of viral

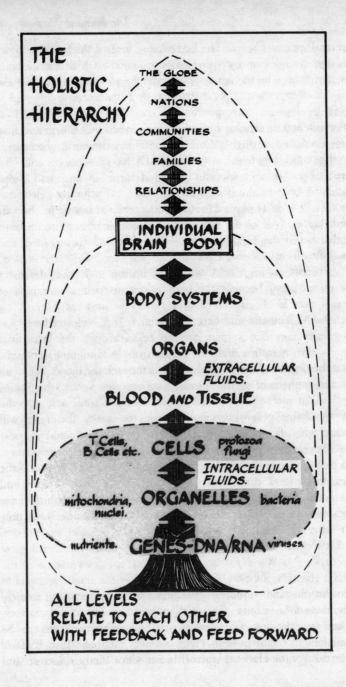

THE HOLISTIC HIERARCHY

THE GLOBE

NATIONS

COMMUNITIES

FAMILIES

RELATIONSHIPS

INDIVIDUAL
BRAIN   BODY

BODY SYSTEMS

ORGANS

EXTRACELLULAR
FLUIDS.

BLOOD AND TISSUE

T Cells,
B Cells etc.   CELLS   protozoa
fungi

INTRACELLULAR
FLUIDS.

mitochondria,   ORGANELLES   bacteria
nuclei.

nutrients.   GENES-DNA/RNA viruses.

ALL LEVELS
RELATE TO EACH OTHER
WITH FEEDBACK AND FEED FORWARD.

research is so time-consuming, difficult and expensive. The result is that they cannot see the breadth and complexity of an individual patient's landscape because of the size of their own particular trees.

Summary

For the person who is severely ill, the healing network may have many fraying meshes. There is a range of possible abnormalities, ranging from the mild to the severe. They are:

- The individual extent of B cell destruction and an ensuing weakening of humoral immunity
- T cell ratio changes affecting cell-mediated immunity
- NK (natural killer) cell reduction reducing protection against herpesviruses and cancer cells
- Red blood cell abnormalities, 'sticky' blood and slower blood flow further weakening the immune defence
- Reduction of neutrophils lessening protection against fungi and bacteria
- Possible viral and fungal crippling of endocrine glands and lymph system
- Smooth muscle antibodies denoting an autoimmune process
- Changes in levels of chemical messengers and hormones
- Interruption of various metabolic processes
- Breakdown of inter-cellular membranes
- Acid/alkaline imbalance and associated energy-using and producing disturbances
- Reduction of intra-cellular RNA

The holes in the mesh still do not entirely explain why some people are ill, and not others; and why some recover quickly, and not others. Diligent seekers after truth, and that includes many people with CFS, know that the truth encompasses far more than the abnormalities that can be seen with the aid of electron microscopes.

THE BRAIN – CONTROL CENTRE

Recent medical research confirms the brain is an important member of the immune network. It is bathed in hormones, chemical messengers linking every nerve in the body, which are triggered by emotions, thought processes and actions. Neurosurgeon Richard Bergland of the Harvard University School of Medicine, says: 'The starting premise of the new knowledge that the brain is a gland is one of unity: the brain is one with the body. Its final observation is one of harmony: hormones come together to do the brain's bidding.'[18] The brain's effect on the immune response is the basis of mysteries such as the placebo effect and recoveries from cancer and chronic diseases. Recently researchers at the National Institute of Mental Health in Maryland and the National Cancer Institute jointly discovered a small molecule, Peptide T, which occurs naturally in the brain. It prevents the AIDS virus from attaching itself to the cells it invades. Scientists even suspect that the brain switches on genes. Brain hormones may move into the very centres of cells and modify the genes controlling them.

William Collinge, who counsels people with immune-related illnesses at Lake Tahoe in Nevada, describes how the brain communicates with the foot soldiers in the immune army. 'Your thoughts and images are transformed into chemical messages (hormones and other substances) by the neurohumoral transducers at the base of your brain. These chemical messages are released into your bloodstream, and they have the effect of telling your immune system what to do. Your immune cells have receptors on their surface, which act like antennae, to receive these messages.'[19]

Messages may even be two-way so that the immune system informs the brain of the type of immune response required, of nutrients that it needs and substances it should avoid. Molecules move not only from the brain to the endocrine system and the body, but also from the endocrine system and other parts of the body to the brain.

'Central to the paradigm that the mind is modulated by hormones is the recognition that the stuff of thought is not caged in the brain, but is scattered all over the body,' Richard Bergland says.[20] This remarkable discovery underlines the dynamic of body-mind interaction and fulfils the holistic paradigms of Eastern philosophy and medicine.

For, as Richard Bergland says, immune mechanisms do not exist in isolation. They are linked by the most exquisite and subtle of networks, powered by hormones, enzymes, and oscillating electrical currents. Our energies respond to the rhythm of words, the phases of the moon and the sounds of music; to beauty and terror, to boredom and challenge, to colour and light.

They respond even to visualisation. They use the results of laboratory tests to show that when a person visualises healthier blood or more vital liver, improvements do follow. Considering the many dreary years during which sufferers of chronic CFS can struggle on, a dreary outlook is not surprising. Thoughts revolve around the weakened body and the processes of degeneration and loss of vitality. Tom O'Connor has kept the AIDS virus at bay through eight years of courage and refusal to accept therapies or experiences which damage immunity. He comments that the subconscious minds of some people with AIDS cannot distinguish between real and imaginary experiences. This results in their being able to feel better simply by using their imaginations.

O'Connor suggests visualisations that blend body and emotion and which take one out of a stifled environment.[21] 'Picture yourself running up a hillside . . . smell the grass, hear the birds singing and your heart beating, taste the sweat running down your face, see the bright blue sky and the puffy white clouds. Visualisations will not only help your body's relaxation mechanisms to mobilise your immunity, but will also help dissolve the blocks to your creative energy, and reprogramme the deep processes of your mind.'

He thinks that people with chronic immune dysfunction should be aware of the energy-draining elements in modern life. He warns against watching gloom, doom and violence on television. A diet of comedy, positivism, classical music and rhyming metred poetry, he says, strengthens the body's energies. O'Connor's advice is as valid for the chronic fatigue syndrome as it is for AIDS.

The importance of these new discoveries cannot be over-emphasised in relation to immune dysfunction illnesses. They legitimise the holistic approach and point to paths that the ill must take in regaining their own health – attention to nutrition, replacement of any negative attitudes, and meditation and spiritual growth.

RECOMMENDED READING:
In Self-Defense, by Stephen B. Mizel and Peter Jaret, Harcourt Brace, 1985. An excellent guide to the workings of the immune system.
Living With AIDS: reaching out, by Tom O'Connor and A. Gonzales-Nunez, Corwin Publishers, San Francisco, 1987.
The Amino Revolution, by Robert Erdmann and Meirion Jones,

Century Hutchinson, 1987.

Man's Search for Meaning, by Viktor E. Frankl, Washington Square Press, 1985.

You Can Heal Your Life, by Louise Hay, Hay House, 1987.

Love, Medicine and Miracles, by Bernie S. Siegel, Harper & Row, 1986.

Your Body Doesn't Lie, by John Diamond, Warner Books, 1979.

Chapter 5   THE IMMUNE NETWORK

1   Duesberg, P.H., 'Retroviruses as carcinogens and pathogens; expectations and reality', *Cancer Research*, 1 March 1987, pp. 1199-220.

2   Valdez, C., Meson, O.E., et al., 'Suppression of humoral response during the course of Candida albicans infection in mice', *Mycopathologica*, 1984, 88:61-3.

3   Saifer, P., 'Endocrinopathy in the Chronic Candidiasis Patient', *Yeast-Human Interaction Symposium*, San Francisco, 1985.

4   Koller, L.D., 'Immunosuppression produced by lead, cadmium and mercury', 1973, *Am.J.Vet.Res.*, 34:11, 1457-8.

5   Draper, M., *Introduction to Food Allergies and Intolerances*, ed. Brostoff, J. and Challacombe, S., Bailliere Tindall 1987.

6   Tuormaa, T.E., 'A Brief Review of the Immune System and its Function in Relation to: PVFS, Non-Antibody Mediated Allergy, Autoimmunity and Immune Deficiency', paper awaiting publication, 1987. Address: Fillebrook, 12 Pixham Lane, Dorking, Surrey RH4 1PT, 9.

7   ibid.

8   ibid.

9   Simpson, L.O., Shand, B.I., Olds, R.J., 'Blood rheology and myalgic encephalomyelitis; a pilot study', *Pathology*, 1986; 18:190-92.

10 Mukherjee, Y., 'Myalgic encephalomyelitis', letter, *Lancet*, 8 August, 1987.

11 Published in the July 1988 periodical of the Medical Research Society (U.K.).

12 Caliguri, M. Cheney, P., et al., 'Phenotypic and functional deficiency of natural killer cells in patients with chronic fatigue syndrome', *Jnl Immunology*, 139, 10, 15 Nov. 1987, pp.3306-13.

13 Undertaken by a team headed by Dr Michael Holmes at Otago Medical School; as yet unpublished.

14 Revici, Emanuel, *Research in Physiopathology as basis of Guided Chemotherapy*. Photocopies of the book are available for US$22.00 from Knowing Business Trust, 8 Muriel Place, Fairfax, California 94930. They also have tapes, books and other material.
15 Communication with author.
16 Revici, Emanuel, 'Research and Theoretical Background for Treatment of the Acquired Immunodeficiency Syndrome (AIDS)', *Townsend Letter For Doctors*, 45, Feb/March 1987.
17 Fowkes, S.W., 'Emanuel Revici, M.E.: novel treatment for heart disease, cancer, AIDS and other chronic diseases', *Jnl Mega Health Society*, 3; 4, July 1987, 1-6.
18 Bergland, Richard, *The Fabric of Mind*, Penguin Books, 1985.
19 Collinge, W., *Activating the healer within; strenthening resistance to immune-related illnesses*, 1987. P.O. Box 3792, Incline Village, Nevada 89450. Counselling courses and additional information available.
20 Bergland, op. cit., pp. 111-21.
21 O'Connor, T. and Gonzalez-Nunez, A., *Living with AIDS – reaching out*, Corwin Publishers, San Francisco, 1987, p.24.

ALLERGIES: FOOD AND CHEMICAL SENSITIVITIES

Many people with chronic illness can be helped. A vast, though still undetermined number of them are suffering from nothing more than a maladaptation to their environment. This maladaptation to corn, wheat, coffee and other common foods, or to natural gas, or to chemical pollutants, is ever-present, ongoing and subtle, so that its nature is rarely even glimpsed by the victim. It is certainly tragic to see such a person shunted from specialist to specialist, none of whom knows any more about his problem than he does – operated upon, maligned, drugged, alienated from friends and family – when all the time his problem was no more mysterious than an intolerance to avoidable foods and chemicals.

THERON G RANDOLPH, MD,
Human Ecology and Susceptibility to the Chemical Environment, 1962.

That food intolerances and chemical sensitivities may underly mysterious intermittent symptoms affecting both brain and body engenders disbelief among most of the medical profession, dietitians and nutritionists. Yet afflicted adults and parents of allergic and hyperactive children know only too well the real nature of their symptoms.

Symptoms particularly associated with hidden allergies include: dizziness, sleepiness, excessive mucus, 'flu-like feelings, asthma, hot flushes, briefly distended veins, inexplicable and sometimes almost immediate weight gain or loss, puffiness (including transitory grotesque swellings of the face), aches and pains in any part of the body, flatulence and bowel disturbances, urinary abnormalities (including bedwetting) . . . the full list is much longer.

Both the traditional medical view and the popular view of food allergies is of some immediate reaction like a rash or swelling experienced after eating strawberries or shellfish. This new hidden type of allergy, more properly called food intolerance or chemical sensitivity, is however, becoming exceedingly common. British immunologist Jonathan Brostoff estimates that about 15 per cent of the population is affected. Clinical ecologists estimate it is the cause for illhealth in about 95 per cent of their patients. The increase in this type of allergy is thought to be due to the increasing number of factors which damage the functioning of the immune system and gut lining. These include viruses, chemicals, stress, immunisation, fungal and parasitical infections and chemical toxins in the body. Intolerance to cow's milk often develops after a viral infection or vaccination, and the gut damage that accompanies cow's milk intolerance may provide a springboard for other food sensitivities.[1]

When chronically ill people consider the possibility that food allergies and intolerances may be at the root of their mystery symptoms, and detect and avoid the culprit foods, they will make a giant step towards regaining health.

Clinical ecologists fear that these allergies are symptomatic of physiological breakdown and represent the thin end of the autoimmune wedge. They worry that the increasing incidence of diseases such as arthritis, lupus, asthma, multiple sclerosis, myasthenia gravis, Crohn's disease, manic-depression, schizophrenia, diabetes and many endocrine disorders is related to this major increase in food and chemical sensitivity.

Food intolerance is now shown to be a 'very substantial' cause of asthma, and should always be considered, especially when it is accompanied by other symptoms. The most common of these are eczema, stomach pains, flatulence and diarrhoea, runny noses and nasal polyps, bedwetting, joint pains, psychological symptoms, urticaria and migraine. Derek Wraith, honorary consultant physician at London's St Thomas' Hospital, writing in the 1987 'allergy bible', *Food Allergy and Intolerance*, edited by British immunologists Drs Jonathan Brostoff and Stephen Challacombe, draws on his own experience and that of many other medical researchers and clinicians to argue this point. He considers that detecting and avoiding the foods in question would prevent much disability and also lessen the quantity of anti-asthma drugs needed – important, considering their expense and potential side effects.[2]

As noted earlier, San Francisco immunologist Allen Scott Levin believes that the cumulative effect of many negative factors in modern life has been to change human physiology and the nature of illness and disease to such an extent that today's doctors are seeing people who are biochemically and genetically different from those of the past. Past case histories and texts are no longer relevant, he says.[3]

In spite of literally hundreds of books and papers on the relationship of hidden allergies to disease, and biochemical research findings going back 30 years or more, the topic of hidden allergies and their almost endless ramifications is still not taught in medical schools or nutritional courses. As a result, drug-oriented psychiatrists and doctors are usually not aware of the effects of food and chemicals on brain and body. Neither are the 'balanced food intake' dietitians or nutritionists.

Thus it is not surprising that most people with the chronic fatigue and immune dysfunction syndrome fail to discover that many of their symptoms are a consequence of what they eat. Their daily bread, dairy products, chocolate, coffee or corn are among the most common foods causing reactions. There are many more. Whatever the food, there will be someone whose body is intolerant to it. New Zealander Sandra Hyder, who now counsels CFS sufferers on diet-related matters, says: 'I remember when a medical specialist, a fellow M.E. sufferer, suggested that our support group in Christchurch should start considering food allergies. I thought he was crazy.'

Prompt attention to diet – removing avoidable burdens from an immune system which is starting to break down – is the best preventive medicine of all. Dr Ricky Gorringe of Cambridge, New Zealand, who has specialised in treating people with immune dysfunction problems, says: 'If someone has only recently acquired

M.E., he or she may have developed an allergy only to wheat, for example. In that case wheat can be eliminated, and the patient go straight on to a rotational diet. If they do not go on to rotation eating, it is as inevitable as night follows day for 95 per cent of them that they will develop further allergies, and they will go down the path of further illhealth.'

Very often foods to which the adult is intolerant are those which were disliked in childhood. Joan, for instance, was upset by cow's milk as a baby and had running battles with her conscientious mother over the daily glass of milk. Joan drank her milk, and gradually came to tolerate it, particularly in chocolate milkshakes. No one connected her frequent headaches and aching legs – or the arthritis that developed in later life – with her regular ingestion of dairy products. Only when Joan developed CFS symptoms in middle-age, and gave up dairy products including the cheese she so loved, did her arthritis disappear along with her more generalised symptoms.

Masked reactions, whether to foods or chemicals, can have marked effects on brain functioning. People commonly report feeling 'spaced out' or removed from reality. Other brain symptoms include depression, migraine, slurred speech, agitation, hyperactivity, irritability, panic attacks and feelings of loss of control. The mechanisms for this are debated. Some specialists believe the cause is allergic reactions in the brain; others point to damaged enzyme systems affecting communication processes; while others point to changed levels of natural chemicals like serotonin and acetycholine.

Abnormal brain activities are so consistent in some people that their ensuing behaviour is thought to be their true nature. This is anything but so. People whose brains are sensitive to the food they eat are truly 'driven' to aggression, violence and irritability. They may have difficulties in reading; their handwriting may be coarse and untidy. They may be baffled, confused and ashamed of what they dimly perceive as an 'uncontrollable being' within them. Episodes leading to court appearances are beginning to be noted. Sensitivities to alcohol and wheat induced such rages in a popular TV personality that he attacked his wife on several occasions. Mental confusion due to eating Twinkie bars was a defence plea for the upright citizen who shot the San Francisco mayor and the alderman Harvey Milk. A Manchester lad who was allergic to potatoes which brought on attacks of uncontrollable behaviour pleaded 'potatoes' in a successful defence of his out-of-character episodes of violence. The young man, his father and defence witness – the clinical ecologist Dr Keith Mumby – were featured on Thames Television in 1984. Clinical ecologists believe that food and chemical sensitivities account for a considerable proportion of the prison population.[4]

There are four ways in which allergenic substances can come in to contact with the body: by direct contact; by injection; by inhalation; and by mouth.

Direct contact

The most obvious one is direct contact on the skin – as with hand lotions, household or industrial liquids, solvents and chemicals, agricultural and horticultural sprays. The hairdresser forced to seek another occupation because of skin reactions to continuous exposure to chemicals is a typical example. There is often an inhalant aspect to contact allergies.

Into the bloodstream

Injections into the bloodstream provide a second avenue for allergen entrance. Susceptible people can have violent, even fatal, allergic direct reactions to drugs injected into their bodies. This is why hospitals now routinely check for allergies to penicillin and other drugs.

Antigens and allergens are now known to be transmitted through body fluids and tissues by such means as blood transfusions and organ and bone-marrow transplants. (Happily, the transplantation of bone-marrow from a non-allergic person can put an end to allergic reactions in the allergic recipient.) Sexual intercourse also carries the possibility of allergy transfers. Body fluids such as semen and saliva have high concentrations of foreign antigens so that multiple different sexual encounters can have the same effects as multiple blood transfusions from different donors.

Inhalant allergens

The inhalant aspect of allergens has probably been underestimated, if the high levels of chemicals found in the noses, throats and lungs of people with chronic fatigue and immune dysfunction are any indication. These are people with disorders in these very areas ... asthma-like symptoms, sore throats, runny noses, puffy and watering eyes, general itching and discomfort in nose and

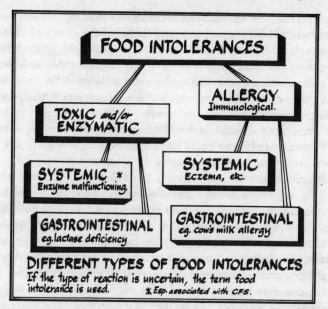

FOOD INTOLERANCES

ALLERGY
Immunological.

TOXIC and/or
ENZYMATIC

SYSTEMIC *
Enzyme malfunctioning.

SYSTEMIC
Eczema, etc.

GASTROINTESTINAL
eg. lactase deficiency

GASTROINTESTINAL
eg. cow's milk allergy

DIFFERENT TYPES OF FOOD INTOLERANCES
If the type of reaction is uncertain, the term food
intolerance is used.   * Esp· associated with CFS.

throat, sore lungs and neurological symptoms. Inhaled allergens
include dust (with dust mites), aromatic odours, animal dander,
moulds and fungal spores, perfumes, hair spray, fly spray, agricultural chemicals and petroleum products.

A severe limitation in the technological age, chemical sensitivity
reduces choice in clothing, furniture and furnishings, cosmetics and
perfumes, household cleansers, paints, varnishes, solvents – and
even employment. The brain is often the organ most affected. As
one example, the incidence of CFS among publishers, editors and
authors is thought by some to be related both to stress and to
frequent exposure to tung oil, found in white correcting fluid and
printing inks.

Sensitivity to petroleum products is more than just a handicap. It
carries a very real public danger. The British clinical ecologist and
psychiatrist Richard Mackarness describes what he calls 'motorway
madness' when people under the influence of petrol fumes lose
their sense of judgement. He comments on the likely outcome with
macho male drivers who are unlikely to admit such a weakness.
Indeed, traffic officers and police often comment on the violent and
half-crazed behaviour of some traffic offenders. Sleepiness and

mental confusion on the road seem more common, however, with members of CFS support groups. Middle-aged Claire said: 'I used to be able to drive for hundreds of miles without feeling tired. Now I start to feel spaced out and fuzzy after 20 miles. My head feels stoned; my eyes start to water and won't work together. So I close one eye, then the other, wiping away the tears – until I have to give up, and pull off the road for a nap.' Claire is now driving long distances again because of her doctor's prescriptions of two drops of Procaine or Heparin under the tongue before she sets off on long trips, with repeats when she feels the symptoms coming on.[5]

People who have experienced petrochemical reactions while driving are convinced that this is a major, unrecognised cause of road accidents, and even of light aircraft accidents. The possibility has not yet been considered, let alone explored, by the medical profession, governments, traffic authorities or transport companies. Many CFS support groups in the United States note an unusually high percentage of members who work at airports or for airlines and are exposed to aviation fuel. As the incidence of CFS rises, the incidence of accidents can be expected to rise.

By way of the mouth

The fourth way the body is exposed to allergens is by way of the mouth and digestive tract. Dr Brostoff summarises what is now known of the subtle and unsuspected ways in which the body protests at foods passing through it. Reactions can be initiated by:

> chemicals in foods, e.g. phenols, caffeine, tyramine;
> salicylate intolerances arising from enzyme defects;
> foods releasing mediators from mast cells;
> irritants to the mucous membranes.

Delayed-type food allergies are confusing because of the ways reactions vary. Four different overlapping types have been identified: addictive, fixed, cumulative and variable. When people suffer withdrawal symptoms if they go without a certain food, that is an **addictive** reaction. When a food has similar and predictable effects on a person, that is a **fixed** reaction. **Cumulative** reactions occur only when the offending food is eaten several times. **Variable** reactions occur when a food affects a person in different ways – a headache one day, a sore throat the next.[6]

Just as with alcoholics and the first drink of the day, many people with CFS frequently feel better after eating their favourite food.

They may feel generally unwell or have marked reactions for a while if they avoid it. Their relationship to that food is one which closely resembles addiction. Those CFS patients who are addicted appear to have more difficulties in regaining control of their bodies than do those without hidden addictions. The medical profession remains generally sceptical.

Chocolate and other food advertisers capitalise on the ups-and-downs of addicted people. They tout their goods as 'a great pick-me-up when you're feeling down'. Those who are addicted know this is true because of the lift they experience after eating or drinking the food in question. If they can't have their chocolate (or tea, coffee, breakfast cereal or soft drink) regularly or on time, symptoms start appearing. It is interesting to contemplate just how much television advertising encompasses the promotion of addiction.

To complicate matters further, sensitivities to any particular foods may not be to the foods themselves but to the chemicals (natural or otherwise) which they contain, or to unsuspected naturally toxic ingredients.[7] Peter, allergic to wheat, could not understand why he reacted to tomato sauce until he realised it was thickened with wheat flour. Home-made muffins were acceptable to Brian, but a major brand of factory-made muffins, with their preservatives, artificial colouring and added enzymes gave him a day in bed.

Clinical ecologists group foods in two ways. The first is into biological families, with particular emphasis on similarity of appearance and physical structure. The second is by naturally occurring constituent chemicals.[8] People who are sensitive to tomatoes, for instance, may be affected by all the foods in the same physical group. These include green peppers, aubergine, potatoes – also tobacco. Or they may be affected by the phenols in tomatoes – or the salicylate, which may give them reactions to salicylates in almonds, chocolate, bananas, berry fruits, garlic, tea, coffee, alcohol – and aspirin. Some salicylate-sensitive people are thought to have acquired this sensitivity through a steady intake of aspirin. Those who are allergic to milk must also suspect all dairy products as well as beef, veal and gelatine, and baked goods and sauces containing milk, butter or cheese. Since cow's milk is high in phenols, they may be phenol-sensitive and must suspect foods with high levels of phenols. People sensitive to sulphites will be affected by many wines and those commercially prepared salads and potato chips where sulphite preparations are used to keep them fresh.

But food sensitivity does not necessarily mean that suspect foods can never be eaten because reactions can be reduced or avoided with a rotation diet. With this diet, foods are eaten in rotation, so that no one particular food is eaten more than once every four days. Highly sensitive people may not be able to eat more than one food from any particular group every four days. A fuller outline of rotational eating is given in the chapter on nutrition, p.177.

Three basic types of allergy are now recognised by clinical ecologists and physicians specialising in immune disorders. Medical traditionalists might not accept these classifications, which have evolved through empirical observations. It should be noted that there are no rigid lines dividing them. Reactions may vary or blur depending on the state of health, stresses and physiological loads – even the weather.

Type 1 Allergies – Immediate

These are the universally accepted shortlived allergic responses to dust, pollens, insect stings and some foods. Patients sneeze and wheeze, cough, scratch, ache and look puffy. Symptoms usually disappear quickly. If there is a systemic reaction, it may result in swelling of tissues and veins, a racing heart, anaphylactic shock, even death. The primary target organs are the nose and respiratory system, the skin, eyes, ears, gastrointestinal tract and occasionally the brain.

These histamine-based immune responses frequently start in infancy or childhood. They often lessen as the years go by. Many well-recognised diagnostic tests and treatments offer a good outlook for Type 1 patients. Those with inherited tendencies or who were colicky as babies are more likely to progress to more serious levels.[9] Some evidence indicates that taking symptom-suppressant drugs which damp down immediate responses may lead to chronic illnesses as in Type 2 allergies and degenerative and autoimmune illnesses as in Type 3 allergies.

Type 2 Allergies – Masked

This is the major CFS type of allergy. It has multiple and often delayed symptoms, often with mood disturbances, chronic fatigue, joint and muscle aches. There is usually a background of loss of immune competency, so that pathogens are not controlled. Type 2 allergies are usually experienced first in hyperactive children, or in adults in their twenties, and affect more women than men. Candida albicans ('thrush') may be a problem and have a causal association with post-natal depression, lumpy breasts, endometriosis and pre-menstrual tension. There are brain reactions such as migraine, confusion, memory loss, personality changes, hyperactivity, sleepiness and depression (often attributed to other causes). Symptoms usually subside when the allergic factor and the candida overgrowth are removed.

Type 2 allergies affect the body generally, but, if they are allowed to continue, immune functioning may deteriorate, enabling further candida albicans overgrowth. As the candida progresses (often helped along by antibiotics taken for ear and sinus infections, cystitis, pneumonia and skin infections) a disease develops, which may eventually become a known entity. It will have a name, affecting a particular organ or body system.[10]

Type 3 Allergies – Autoimmune
Autoimmunity is when people are not only allergic to elements in their external environment, but also become allergic to themselves, perhaps to specific organs, enzymes, hormones or to the candida overgrowths in their bodies. Any allergic reaction against internal fungal infestations will damage the organs involved. This is the level at which autoimmune diseases develop. The endocrine glands, particularly the thyroid, thymus and adrenals, are especially threatened. They literally shrivel under the stress of the antibody-antigen overload, direct fungal effects and other factors in immune dysfunction blockage. Antibodies to their own brains have been detected in the bodies of schizophrenics and autistic children.

Some organ-specific autoimmune diseases associated with Type 3 allergies are: thyroiditis (thyroid); Addison's disease (adrenals); oophoritis (PMS and premature ovarian failure) and female reproductive problems; alopecia; pituitary disease; insulin dependent diabetes; pernicious anaemia; vitiligo; myasthenia gravis; pemphigus; chronic biliary cirrhosis and progressive hepatitis; schizophrenia and autism.

THE INSIDE STORY
Many complex biochemical and physiological processes take place as sensitivities, intolerances and allergies develop. All create their own problems which may be difficult to detect, let alone correct. The most important are changes in the body's pH (acid/alkaline level); rising deposits of cholesterol and distortions and stiffenings of both the red blood cells and lymphocytes; alterations in hormone production; and fluctuating blood sugar levels leading to diabetes-like symptoms. These blood sugar fluctuations often precede the development of allergies, and are part and parcel of the allergic experience. Antibody and histamine reactions take place in the histamine-producing mast cells in the gut, connective tissues, organs, endocrine glands and various cells in the blood, including platelets.

All types of allergies have faulty T cell functioning in common. Reduced suppressor T cell activity and overactive B cells are found in Type 1 allergies. This produces an overload of an antibody called IgE (immunoglobulin E). In Type 2 allergies, underactive suppressor T cells and a different kind of B cell produce a different kind of antibody known as IgG (immunoglobulin G). Particularly in allergy types 2 and 3, the function of T cells and all cells and all body processes are affected by enzyme dysfunction.

Enzymes are the catalysts of the body, enabling the body to carry out its functions, maintain its tissues and digest food. Many thousands of these proteins are produced, each interacting with others and with vitamins (co-enzymes) or minerals enabling energy release and metabolic processes to take place. Abnormal activity levels in one enzyme pathway will lead to alterations in others, since all are inter-related. An enzyme may be present, but may be so underactive that toxic products build up. Enzymes are responsible for the processing of everything that is required by the body for life – for thought, for movement, for digestion. Enzymes are also crucial in processing everything that the body needs to get rid of to retain life. One single enzyme deficiency can disrupt critical processes. If the deficiency is major and permanent, it will lead to a gradual deterioration in liver, muscle and brain, and, quite possibly, death.

Long-term nutritional deficiencies affect the functioning of the particular enzymes to which they relate. Stressed metabolic pathways due to abnormal enzyme functioning are thought to explain why food intolerances fluctuate. They are a principal reason why rotational eating and the eight-on-a-plate approach (see Chapter 13) are so helpful. American clinical ecologist Dr William Philpott observes, for instance, that a person with an enzymatically disordered urea cycle metabolism and with carnosine or anserine intolerance would have reactions from a meal that included a large helping of red meat (containing carnosine and anserine). That same person would be symptom-free with a much smaller helping of meat. The big helping could overstress the enzyme's capacity for digestion, leaving large protein molecules to be absorbed into the body, causing inflammatory reactions.[11]

Jonathan Brostoff suggests that people with allergies and intolerances are, in general, poor metabolisers, and that a double defect, such as an enzyme weakness and an immune response gene can make an individual very susceptible to food allergens and chemicals.[12] Such a link is that provided by the HLA-B8 genetic marker which increases susceptibility to adrenal and thyroid disorders, chronic hepatitis, myasthenia gravis, arthritis, lupus and gluten sensitivity. There will be hereditary weaknesses in similar enzyme functioning in all those individuals carrying that marker.

Britain's Dr Keith Mumby, who specialises in allergies and CFS, says, 'One thing we do know about enzymes is that they poison easily – even trace amounts of the wrong thing can stop them working. Interference with enzyme systems will lead to a greater intolerance of other chemicals. Foods are basically chemicals and are digested by enzymes – different ones for fats, starches, sugar, proteins and so on. It is to be expected that an inability to deal properly with foods is a consequence of the widespread presence in the environment of toxic substances.'[13]

CFS researchers have found many specific enzyme deficiencies, enough to raise the thought that the syndrome's most significant feature may be of multiple enzyme deficiencies. These include adenylate deaminase[14] and adenosine diphosphate,[15] both of which are involved in muscle energy processes. Dr Peter Behan draws parallels between the post viral syndrome and Reyes Syndrome in which mitochondrial abnormality in muscle tissue is thought to be the essential cause, and illnesses caused by carnosine intolerance and arginine deficiency.[16] Dr Melvin Ramsay, the 'father' of M.E. research, noted several enzyme abnormalities, including GOT,

GPT, and *r*-glutamyl transferase. Some are similar to those in muscular dystrophy, others to those in liver damage.[17] Canadian researcher Irving Salit found abnormal levels of 2,5-oligo-adenylate synthetase in most CEBV patients.[18] This is a marker for interferon.

Dr Belinda Dawes, an Australian clinical ecologist now practising in London, sees many patients with deficiencies of pyridoxyl phyphosphatase (essential in vitamin B6 metabolism), delta 6-desaturase (involved in Omega 6 fatty acid pathways) and DNA RNA transferase, an enzyme which has a requirement for zinc. 'One good thing,' she says, 'is that antioxidant enzyme systems are normal in most of my patients. These are the predisposing factors in aging and cancer.'

An important enzyme deficiency in chronic fatigue syndrome patients is attributed by Trowbridge and Walker to candida overgrowth. 'Many people victimised by candidiasis cannot process essential fatty acids efficiently. Candida toxin . . . gets absorbed into the bloodstream and carried right throughout the body. It interferes with an enzymatic protein that is a vital processor of long-chain fatty acids, important in maintaining membranes, in conducting metabolism, and in producing local hormones called prostaglandins,' they write in *The Yeast Syndrome*.[19]

Deficiencies of what is probably the same enzyme, delta-6-desaturase, is found in salicylate sensitivity. The fatty acid/prostaglandin pathway is more easily inhibited by salicylates in individuals with salicylate sensitivity. The *Medical Journal of Australia* reported in 1984[20] that more systemic reactions occurred with salicylates than with any other food constituent. This perhaps reflects the very high Australian intake of aspirin. A new Australian version of the Feingold diet for hyperactive children features the avoidance of all foods containing salicylates. New Zealander Patricia Holborow, who carried out nine years' research with salicylate-sensitive children in Queensland, describes widespread allergic reactions, hyperactivity, night terrors and problems with study. These were corrected by the avoidance of salicylates. She also provides a visual diagnosis for salicylate-sensitive children. In addition to puffiness, particularly around the eyes, there may be a red weal (resembling windburn) or a rash under the lower lip.

Holborow has a particular interest in the links between cot death and salicylate sensitivity. She believes that any marked variation in quantities and regularity of salicylate-containing foods (such as orange juice, at a time when a salicylate-sensitive baby's immune system and respiratory centre are under stress, as for instance, if it has a cold, may be the cot death trigger.[21] Her recommendations reflect findings from many sources.

THE COT DEATH CONNECTION

Sudden Infant Death syndrome, SIDS, research elsewhere has come up with other enzyme deficiencies linking liver damage and cot deaths. Sheffield University's cot death research team found deficiencies of an enzyme known as medium-chain-acetylcozyme-A dehydrogenase in up to 7 per cent of cot deaths in the 200 cases they studied.[22] As with delta series desaturases, this deficiency leads to an inability to metabolise certain fatty acids. The fatty changes in the livers of those babies were similar to those in the livers of children with Reye's syndrome, a disease linked with aspirin and salicylate sensitivity. 'One in four siblings of a cot death baby will be at risk of inheriting the disorder. We think it important that if a family has had a cot death, subsequent babies should be tested for the enzyme defect in the neonatal period,' said Alec Howat, as reported in *New Scientist* in 1986. He said that if one enzyme deficiency had been identified as a contributing factor in some cot deaths, perhaps other similar defects might be responsible. 'There are thousands of enzymes in the body. Why should others not cause cot deaths, too?'

Other enzyme deficiencies have indeed been implicated in cot deaths. They include biotinidase, galactase and enzymes responsible for metabolising ammonia,[23] and vitamin E, iron and selenium.[24]

The latter study, by Donald Money of New Zealand's Wallaceville Animal Research Centre, found significantly lower levels of vitamin E and selenium and higher levels of iron in the livers of 120 cot death babies than in the 17 livers from children who had died from other causes. The enzyme involved, glutathione peroxidase, GTP, helps remove pollutants from the body. It is an important anti-oxidant and anti-cancer enzyme, preventing oxygen from reacting with other substances and damaging cells. This 'free radical' reaction is enhanced by surplus iron. Problems with iron metabolism were noted by Campbell Murdoch in his 1986 study of people with M.E.

These enzyme abnormalities are similar to those found in various inherited diseases, diseases which have been recorded for centuries. They bring to mind the inability of various ancient Greeks, among them Pythagoras, to metabolise fava beans because of an inherited lack of the enzyme glucose-6-phosphate dehydrogenase (or G-6-PD), and the present campaign by some Mediterranean health authorities to test blood donors for this condition because it can be transferred by blood transfusions. Today there are growing numbers of unhappy children forced to live in space suits or plastic bubbles because of their 'intolerance to the modern world'. These children lack the immune system enzyme adenosine deaminase (ADA).

Medical literature now abounds with reports of chemically-caused outbreaks of CFS-type disease related to enzyme breakdown. They illustrate the thin line between chemical poisoning and allergic reactions, in that allergic reactions are said to be responses that do not occur in most people. But when people are malnourished, or have immune deficiencies, their defences are obviously weaker. An example is that of the 3,000 Turkish children who developed porphyria during the years 1955–9 after eating seed wheat treated with a fungicide containing hexachlorobenzene. Around 300 died. Those who became ill were generally undersized and undernourished.[25] Twenty-five years later, most of the original victims were still ill, with all organs and especially the liver being affected and high levels of hexachloro-benzene being measured in blood. Many were less affected. Later studies suggested damage to metabolic processes involving the amino acid glycine. Porphyria is an enzyme-related disease with symptoms that bear many similarities to those of CFS. Chelation therapy with EDTA (see glossary) used intravenously proved to be the most helpful treatment for the Turkish sufferers.[26] Hexachlorobenzene, with a three-year half-life, is one of the most dangerous agricultural chemicals known, and is now banned in most countries.

Widespread porphyria-type outbreaks are reported in domestic and wild animals exposed to chemicals (particularly hexachlorobenzene). High levels of this fungicide, widely used for the control of rusts and moulds in cereals and horticulture, were found in the body fat of Australians in 1972.[27] In Japan, 15,000 people developed porphyria in 1968 after eating PCB-contaminated rice oil.[28]

These examples illustrate the sliding scale of chemical burdens in the body, with low sub-toxic levels at one end which may be sufficient to tip the body into sensitivity. That first sensitivity usually shows up in intolerances to substances containing phenol or to alcohol, giving a warning to those who suddenly find liquor disagrees with them. As chemical overloads from whatever source increase, so does immune dysfunction and enzyme damage leading to organ dysfunction and even death.

New Zealand's Campbell Murdoch puts it another way, seeing health and a pure environment at one end of the scale, with growing burdens of toxic chemicals building up through allergic reactions to organ dysfunction and even breakdown at the other end. His view is shared by Dr Douglas Seba of Washington, D.C., medical researcher and specialist in the health effects of toxic chemicals, and former scientific adviser to the United States Environmental Protection Agency, who says: 'Most medical work has been in the area of organ dysfunction. Once you have a diseased liver, gall bladder or whatever, then your disease has a name and they can cut it out. What we are concerned with is what is happening before it becomes a fixed disease.'

Dr Seba believes that the chemical overload in people's bodies is the fundamental cause of widespread illhealth related to immune disorders and weakness. He argues that the most important danger in repeated low-level exposures is the problem of chemical build-up. The accumulation of a chemical in the body is dependent on three factors: the dose, the dose interval and the half-life of the chemical. A chemical with a short half-life can be rapidly eliminated, but if its half-life is long, the body burden never returns to zero.[29] The individual ability to metabolise chemicals is another major factor, with the health of enzymes and liver being of prime importance.

There is special concern at possible reductions in cholinesterase levels caused by organophosphates such as Malathion, Diazinon and Parathion. This enzyme switches off the production of the chemical messenger acetylcholine after messages have been sent. The table indicates the integral role acetylcholine plays in body functioning, and the various symptoms associated with its damage.[30] While some symptoms may pass in a few hours, subtle, delayed and permanent effects on brain functioning may also occur. Damage to other enzymes may be permanent. Organophosphates are by no means the only agricultural culprits in neurological damage. Others include the carbamates (Carbaryl); chlorinated hydrocarbons (DDT, Aldrin, Dieldrin, Chlordane, Heptachlor, etc.); and other pesticides, fumigants (such as methyl bromide) and solvents.

ACETYLCHOLINE AND PESTICIDES

Function of nerves that are stimulated by acetylcholine	Effect of excessive stimulation caused by carbamate or organophosphate pesticides
Activate salivary, sweat, tear glands	Increased salivation, sweating, watering of eyes
Constrict bronchi	Tightness in chest, bronchospasms, difficulty breathing
Contract pupil of eye	Pin-point pupils, blurring of vision
Control heart function	Abnormal heart beat, change in blood pressure
Increase spasms in digestive tract	Stomach cramps, nausea, vomiting, diarrhea
Increase spasms in urinary tract	Urinary frequency and incontinence
Activate skeletal muscles	Twitching, restlessness, tremulousness, impaired

	coordination, general muscle weakness, paralysis
Alter brain function	Headache, giddiness, anxiety, emotional instability, lethargy, confusion, and eventually severe central nervous system depression and coma.

Reprinted from *Journal of Pesticide Reform*, Summer 1986

Thus the allergy epidemic, thought by many dieticians and medical professionals to be hysterical or psychosomatic,[31] is understandable when it is viewed as an indication of a general lessening of immune competency. The example of the Turkish children explains why, given the same physical trauma, even the same genetic background, some people become allergic because of their poor physical state, while others are not affected. Today, in the midst of plenty, affluent people are frequently malnourished, with vitamin and trace element deficiencies and digestive and metabolic disorders caused by too much sugar, refined carbohydrates and chemical additives, and too little fresh foods and natural fibre in the diet. Others are unable to absorb all the vitamins and minerals from what appear to be well-balanced diets.

A California dental researcher, Dr Francis Pottenger, ran a three-generation research programme on cats, comparing the health of those fed on raw meat, natural milk and cod-liver oil with those fed on cooked meat and pasteurised milk. At the end of the second generation the first group of cats was healthy, happy and fertile. The second was asthmatic, arthritic, allergic, bad-tempered, infertile. There was no third generation for the 'cooked meat cats'. An alarming aspect was that the cats taken off the deficient diet then took three generations to return to normal health levels.[32]

Dr Keith Mumby considers that Pottenger's findings are important to today's proliferation of chronic diseases in humans: 'parallels with our modern human diets are inevitable, and if the findings hold true for us as well as for cats the implications are very serious indeed: namely that through bad eating we are ruining not only our own health but also that of our children and grandchildren.'[33]

For information about allergy treatments and methods of detoxification, see Chapters 12 and 13.

Summary:

1. Allergies and intolerances are organic disorders, are extremely complex and affect every system of the body.
2. Heredity, environment and infections, particularly viruses, are causative factors in all types of allergies.
3. The sliding scale of metabolic breakdown stretches from vague symptoms and intolerances to organ dysfunction and death.
4. The availability of a wide range of enzyme tests for patients with intransigent symptoms is essential.
5. Intolerances caused by enzyme dysfunction can usually be corrected by nutritional supplementation to boost the particular metabolic pathway, together with rotational eating.
6. The association between cot deaths, enzyme deficiencies and the chronic fatigue and immune dysfunction syndrome needs to be researched thoroughly.

A CHECKLIST OF ALLERGY-RELATED SYMPTOMS AND COMPLAINTS

Respiratory problems: asthma and wheezing; runny or itching noses; recurrent nosebleeds; bronchitis. Often accompanied by red, runny eyes.

Skin: eczema; rashes and hives; urticaria; persistent itches and soreness; dermatitis; mouth ulcers.

Digestive system: diarrhoea; irritable bowel syndrome; colitis; ulcers; vomiting; gallstones.

Head: migraines; sinus headaches; muscle-tension headaches after food; facial swelling.

Ears: ringing or buzzing, blocked; sounds too loud or too soft; intermittent hearing loss.

Mind: emotions and nervous system; depression and manic-depression; aggressive behaviour and irritability; lethargy; panic attacks; difficulty in concentrating; hyperactivity (especially in children); giddiness; convulsions.

Genito-urinary: bedwetting; frequent urination; cystitis; recurrent thrush.

Muscles and joints: aches and pains for no apparent reason;

sometimes excruciating back pains in association with other muscle and joint aches.

Heart and circulation: pulse that races after any particular food; pains that are mistaken for angina or heart attacks; high blood pressure; migraine; blushing or blanching for no reason.

RECOMMENDED READING

Brain Allergies: the psycho-nutrient connection, by Wm H. Philpott and Dwight K. Kalita, Keats Publishing Inc., U.S. 1980. A vital resource for the health professional and informed lay person.

Allergies, Your Hidden Enemy, by Theron G. Randolph and Ralph Moss, Turnstone Press, U.K. 1981. One of the most important books on allergies by one of the most important clinical ecologists. Suitable for both professionals and lay readers. Includes food families.

Diet, Crime and Delinquency, by Alexander Schauss, Parker House, Berkeley, U.S. Demonstrates how food allergies, junk foods and lead poisoning can foster violence. Brief studies. Good bibliography.

Food, Mind and Mood, by David Sheinkin, Michael Schacter and Richard Hutton, Warner Books, U.S., 1979. Highlights the concepts of energy flow as related to brain sensitivities and testing. Food families and sample menus.

The Allergy Relief Programme: Type 1 and Type 2, by Alan S. Levin and Merla Zellerbach, Gateway Books, 1983. An outstanding self-help guide. Food families included.

The Food Allergy Plan, by Keith Mumby, Unwin Paperbacks, London, 1985. Practical and straightforward guide to self-help.

Allergy Overload: Are Foods and Chemicals Killing You? by Stephen Griffiths, Fontana, 1987. Excellent coverage of the Australian scene and reference to M.E.

Food Intolerance and How to Cope With It, by Robert Buist, Harper & Row, Australia, 1984. Highly recommended.

Dr Mandell's 5-day Allergy Relief System, by Marshall Mandell and L.W. Scanlon, Arrow Books, U.K., 1983. Highly recommended, far thinking, with dietary and environmental programmes, charts and questionnaires.

Not All In The Mind, by Richard Mackarness, Pan, London, 1976. A psychiatrist looks at the role of food and chemical allergens in psychiatric and mental symptoms. Highly recommended.

Chemical Victims, by Richard Mackarness, Pan, London. 1980. Focusses on the role of sub-toxic exposures to chemicals in immune dysfunction.

Food For Thought, by Maureen Minchin, Alma Publications, Melbourne, 1982. A guide to feeding infants and children so as to avoid the development of allergies.

Food Allergy and Intolerance, ed. Jonathon Brostoff and Stephen Challacombe, Bailliere Tindall, 1987. This 1032-page volume is a compendium of the latest research on basic mechanisms of food allergy, food components and their effects, diagnostic methods and treatments. Contributions from world figures in established medicine and clinical ecology.

Chapter 6 ALLERGIES

1 Gerard, J.W., 'Cow's Milk and Breast Milk', in Brostoff, J.A. and Challacombe, S., eds., *Food Allergy and Intolerance*, Bailliere Tindall, London, 1987.

2 Wraith, D.G., 'Asthma', in Brostoff, J.A., and Challacombe, S., eds., *Food Allergy and Intolerance*, Bailliere Tindall, London, 1987, pp.486-97.

3 Levin, A.S. and Zellerbach, M., *The Allergy Relief Programme*, Gateway Books, 1983, pp.21-4.

4 Schauss, A., *Diet, Crime and Delinquency*, Parker House, Berkeley, California, 1981.

5 The suggestion came from Philpott, W.H. and Kalita, D.K. *Brain Allergies: the psycho-nutrient connection*, Keats Pub. Co., 1980, p.46. Homoeopaths use homoeopathic petroleum preparations for the same purpose.

6 Brostoff, J., 'Mechanisms: an introduction', in *Food Allergy and Intolerance*, 1987, pp.433-55.

7 Natural toxic substances are found in minute quantities in many foods. They include phenols (found in beef, cabbage, chicken and eggs, potato and tomato); histamine (found in cheese, wine, most tinned foods, tomato); salicylates; caffeine; tannin; rutin, gallic acid, and other chemicals; aflatoxins; oxalates; muscarin; and protease inhibitors. Cow's milk is particularly high in naturally occurring toxins, particularly phenols. Lectins, which affect blood agglutination, are found in several varieties of beans, in tomatoes, peas, lentils and wheatgerm.

8 Levin, A.S. and Zellerbach, M., op. cit., pp.34-58.

9 ibid, pp.59-88.

10 Saifer, P.L. & Becker, N., 'Allergy and autoimmune endocrinopathy; APICH syndrome', in *Food Allergy and Intolerance*, 1987, pp. 781-96.

11 Philpott, W.H. and Philpott, K., 'Principles of Bio-Ecologic Medicine', *Jnl Orthomolecular Psychiatry*, 11, 3, 208-15.

12 Brostoff, J. op cit., p.445.

13 Mumby, K., *The Food Allergy Plan*, Unwin Paperbacks, 1985, p.42.

14 Staines, E., 'Myalgic encephalomyelitis hypothesis', *Med. Jnl. Aust.*, 143, 22 July 1985. Describes disruption of the purine nucleotide cycle through adenylate deaminase deficiency.

15 Behan, P.O., Behan, W.H. and Bell, E.J., 'The post-viral syndrome – an analysis of the findings in 50 cases', *Jnl Infection*, 1985, 10, 211-22.

16 ibid.

17 Ramsay, A.M. & Rundle, A., 'Clinical and biochemical findings in ten patients with benign myalgic encephalomyelitis', *Postgrad. Med. Jnl*, Dec 1979, 55, 856-7.

18 Salit, I.E., 'Sporadic postinfectious neuromyasthenia', *Can Med Asso Jnl*, 133, 659-63.

19 Trowbridge, J.P. and Walker, M., *The Yeast Syndrome*, Bantam, 1986, pp.169-70.

20 *Medical Jnl. Aust*, Sept, 1 1984, Special Supplement.

21 Holborow, P., 'Sudden Infant Death Syndrome' (letter), *Am. Jnl Clinical Nutrition*, 1980, Apr. 33(4) 730-1.

22 Robertson, H. 'Cot deaths linked to faulty enzyme', *New Scientist*, 18 Sept. 1986, p.31.

23 Tyler, J.W., *Sudden Infant Death; Probable Causes and Simple Prevention*, 1986, Sterling Publishing, N.Y., and Reed Methuen, N.Z.

24 Money, D.F.L., 'Vitamin E., selenium, iron and vitamin A content of livers from Sudden Infant Death Syndrome cases and control children; Interrelationships and possible significance', *N.Z. Jnl Science*, 1978, 21:41-55.

25 Strik, J.J.T.W., 'Porphyrinogenic action of polyhalogenated aromatic compounds, with special reference to Porphyria and environmental impair', in *Int. Symposium of Clinical Biochemistry, Diagnosis and Therapy of Porphyrias and Lead Intoxication*, ed. M. Doss, 1978, Springer Verlag. This Dutch toxologist argues that the accumulation of porphyrins in the livers of those exposed to chemicals leads on through liver damage to acquired porphyria.

26 Peter, H.A. et al., *Am. Jul Med. Sci.*, 1966, 251, 104.

27 Brady, M.N. and Siyali, D.S., 'Hexachlorobenzene in human body fat', *Med Jnl Aust.*, 22 Jan 1972, 158-61.

28 Umeda, G., 'PCB poisoning in Japan', *Ambio 1*, 1972, 132-4.
29 Seba, D.B., Milam, M.J. and Laseter, J.L., 'Uptake, measurement and elimination of synthetic chemicals by man', in *Food Allergy and Intolerance*, 1987, pp.401-15.
30 Young, B.B., 'Neurotoxicity of pesticides', *Jnl Pesticide Reform*, Summer 1986, 6:2, 8-10.
31 Pearson, D.J., 'Pseudo food allergy', *BMJ* 25 Jan 1986, 282:6515, 221-2.
32 Pottenger, F., *Pottenger's Cats – a study in nutrition*, Price-Pottenger Nutrition Foundation, 1983. Part 2 is concerned with human nutrition.
33 Mumby, op. cit., pp.34-5.

A RANGE

OF CASE HISTORIES

Wide differences in ages, backgrounds and philosophies mark these personal stories, but all have the common ground of apparently inexplicable fatigue together with varied and fluctuating symptoms illustrative of the chronic fatigue and immune dysfunction syndrome. Those affected by chemicals show a higher degree of environmental sensitivity than do those for whom persistent viruses were involved. These examples also indicate how treatments differ both in their approach and their effectiveness.

CARLA – Candida and Homoeopathy

Carla, an American in her 30s, has been a television reseacher, programme-planner and news reader. She still hopes to become a producer, but when she gave this interview she was far from well after eight years of illness, and had been suspended from her job.

'When I look back on my early life, I realise I was never really well. My appendix burst when I was nine, and I always seemed to be on penicillin for tonsilitis. Hay fever began when I was 13, and my stomach became swollen and painful. I think now that this was the start of my candida problem. How I hated school lunches! Whenever I could, I ate mostly bread and cheese.

'As far back as I can remember, I've seemed to have a peculiar feeling as if I were fermenting. If I ate apples, I'd get as high as if I were drunk, and all my life I've got high on fruit juices, with or without sugar. That's why I never drink alcohol.'

After graduation Carla worked in Italy for a few years, on an English-language paper and on the Voice of America. Italy, 'not as cold and damp as at home', made her feel more energetic and capable.

Back home, she was deeply involved in a television career, 'with doors beginning to open for me', when she became severely ill in 1980 with what was thought to be bronchitis, but what she now knows to have been a viral influenza, the trigger for her chronic fatigue syndrome.

Her doctor gave her antibiotics, course after course. 'Each time I'd feel worse, with attacks of cystitis, and what I now realise was rampant candida. After almost two months I knew I'd have to get back to work or I'd be crowded off the career ladder. I remember saying to that docotor, "I must be better but I don't feel it".'

Bloating, dizziness and fatigue continued. Noise and bright lights began to bother her. Another doctor prescribed a course of anti-thrush medication, but said nothing at all about diet. 'Please, what's wrong with me?' she asked, but there was no answer.

Desperate to get better, Carla asked for second opinions. One doctor said she needed to get married and have a baby. A consultant asked her what she herself thought was the problem. When she tentatively suggested allergies, he said, 'There is no such thing as allergies.' Then he recommended a psychologist. Carla wondered how symptoms such as her swollen body and cystitis could be psychosomatic. She became worse.

'In the office everyone thought I was a clown. I had to read and check all the newspapers but I couldn't take in what I read. My brain wouldn't function. I forgot names. I couldn't read my VDU so couldn't see my mistakes – words would blur. My spelling and grammar were all shot. The others would laugh behind my back. My own words were back to front. I remember saying, 'That's a nice black tablecloth.' It was white. And I'd stutter and couldn't finish sentences.

'I felt as if I couldn't get enough air for my brain to work. My brain seemed like a thick velvet curtain at a theatre, with someone (me) trying to get through.'

The next time Carla collapsed, she was in bed for seven weeks. 'By then my boss wanted to get rid of me. When I dragged myself back to the office, I was made to work non-stop through Christmas and New Year, doing routine chores. I begged others to check my work for errors because I couldn't see them. Then I saw not very bright people doing my work better than I could – it was soul-destroying. I'd always been an ideas person. Now I was too ill to carry an idea through.

'The shifts in the TV newsroom were long, 1-11 p.m. or 8 a.m.-6 p.m. I just couldn't get out of bed for an 8 a.m. start. I was exhausted. After 11 p.m. they'd send me home in a taxi. I'd stumble into bed, then stumble out of bed for work by 1 p.m. again.

'The network's own doctor kept saying, "Stress. She's in her 30s and no baby." I was too feeble even to pick up somebody else's baby . . . My mother, a senior social worker, kept telling doctors that I was physically ill, but they didn't believe her, either.'

Carla was determined to find out what was wrong, get herself better, and get on with her career and a normal life. 'I nagged my GP into referring me to the allergy department of a hospital. There I met a cruel doctor. She asked me my symptoms, then interrupted me and said I needed a psychiatrist. I thought that might help – in spite of the doctor's sarcasm – as by then I was carrying a load of anger about my illness and the way doctors were treating me. But I'd arranged a holiday in Mexico so went there first. Amazingly, in the heat and dryness of Mexico my symptoms seemed to clear up. Sightseeing made me tired, but it was an ordinary healthy tiredness.'

Back at work in the United States, her symptoms returned. She went again to the 'cruel doctor' who this time prescribed laxatives as well as urging psychiatric help. Carla by now was so convinced that any emotional problems were because of her physical illness that she parted company with this doctor.

Now ill for nearly five years, Carla in desperation went to a homoeopathic clinic. 'There a wonderful old man saw me. In just seven minutes he said, "My poor dear – you have a very bad case of candidiasis." He recommended books on candida albicans overgrowth, and told me what foods to avoid and what vitamin supplements to take, and offered to give me free vitamin B injections.

'Most of all, this old homoeopathic doctor listened to me. He believed me. He saved my life. When he said I'd got candida, for the first time in front of any doctor I cried, with relief. He put his arms around me – the old darling.'

He wrote a letter for her to give the network doctor who didn't know about candida and wouldn't believe in it. Carla's attempts to describe candida's effects on the body met with anger and further insistence that she needed psychiatric help. The upshot was being summoned to the television channel's personnel department, 'and ticked off for upsetting our doctor'.

The homoeopathic doctor followed up by sending photocopied information on candida to the network doctor, then another anxious letter, which resulted in Carla's being referred for blood tests at a medical school hospital. There she was told she was suffering from chronic Epstein-Barr virus. 'Being told something definite was such a relief, even if they said there was nothing they could do for me.'

Carla's mother paid for her to join a private health scheme. Carla disclosed details of the virus and knew she couldn't claim for illness related to chronic Epstein-Barr as she must have had it for some time. Then an allergist whom she visited because of intensifying illness told her he thought she should be tested for allergies at a private hospital covered by her health insurance. There Carla was tested and told she had multiple allergies. She struggled to follow directions regarding her diet, but 'almost went into shock' when she was faced with a huge hospital bill. The private insurance scheme had refused to pay.

'People should be extremely careful to check the fine print of any health insurance policy. There was a clause in mine saying that if you had a disease when you joined the scheme – even if you didn't know about it – you wouldn't be eligible for insurance payments. And they claimed I must have had allergies all the time.'

Carla now follows a careful anti-candida diet. She avoids foods she is particularly sensitive to and practises rotational dieting, leaving a four-day interval before again eating a particular food or food family. She supplements her diet with vitamins and minerals prescribed by her new doctor, and says that the past year of her eight-year illness has brought a gradual but perceptible improvement in her health. She does not know when she will be able to return to work, and she is still haunted by the debt she owes to the private hospital. – CCC

FRED – Rest and Vitamin C

Fred, a New Zealand farmer in his late 40s, is pale, gaunt, and feels wretched most of the time. He has lost about 28 pounds in weight since he became ill in 1978 during the initial M.E. outbreak in Otago. His doctor sent samples of his blood to the Pasteur Institute in Paris in 1981 but no virus or any specific abnormalities were found. Initially it was thought he might have hepatitis because of liver abnormalities.

Fred describes the chronic fatigue syndrome as wrecking his health, just as it is ruining his life. 'Sometimes I feel so depressed and so mentally confused that I have begged to be committed to a mental hospital. My legs ache nearly all the time. Sometimes they burn – or they tingle. I have terrible sweats about once a fortnight. Urinating is sometimes like passing blocks of concrete.'

Fred developed a number of food intolerances. These include meat, which makes him vomit, and cooked tomatoes. He is able to continue working, though at a less strenuous level, by taking plenty of rest and large amounts of vitamin C (up to 30 grammes daily).He is still not well; has not had his food intolerances identified; nor has he followed any thorough detoxification programme.

Fred lives in a rural area, heavily fertilised with superphosphate and heavily sprayed with agricultural chemicals. There are marked soil deficiencies, particularly of selenium, iodine and manganese. There is a high incidence of stock diseases including spontaneous abortion in sheep, scabby mouth and white muscle disease. All these are related to viruses and trace element deficiencies.

JAN – Nutrition and Avoidance of Allergens

A middle-aged critical care nurse in the United States, devoted to her work and family, Jan became ill in 1986. She had a history of minor allergies and chest compaints, and a candida problem, as she now recognises.

Jan has become extremely sensitive to foods and chemicals, so much so that she and her husband left their Los Angeles home to live in a mountain cabin which they are trying to make completely 'safe' or non-allergenic. She asks visitors not to wear perfume, scented cosmetics or after-shave lotion and this interview was given in the open air.

'I was in the middle of my busy life when I came down with pneumonia early in 1986, and was given the usual antibiotics. Although I recovered I couldn't shake off an extraordinary fatigue. My heart rate was high, but a cardiologist couldn't find anything wrong. I developed bronchitis and asthma, and had more medications.

'A few months later the hot water heater in our home flooded, and our synthetic carpet was saturated. The insurance company brought in giant fans to dry the place, and they blew out fumes, mould, mildew – their effect was unbelievably horrible. Twice I had to be taken to the emergency room. A conventional allergist did 80 scratch tests and I nearly collapsed. "No more invasive tests," I said.'

Jan went from doctor to doctor, trying to find someone who would help. The response was always along these lines: 'We can't find any reason. Therefore your illness must by psychological.' She was sure this was not so in that her personal, family and working lives were completely happy, except for her illness.

'I wish doctors weren't worried about loss of face. Most doctors don't understand environmental illness because they didn't learn about it when they trained. Most don't like to say, "I don't know what's wrong with you, but I believe you when you say there *is* something wrong." I expect they can't believe unless they know the patient very well. This gets to be so hurtful. It isn't "all in your head".'

Jan began reading books on allergies and realised she had developed chemical sensitivities as well as food allergies. She had also become sensitive to electromagnetic impulses in that she felt worse when exposed to household appliances such as a television set or washer-dryer.

Electroacupuncture and rotation dieting (on a very limited number of foods) have helped her. Expert nutritional care with supplements of vitamins and minerals is essential, she says. Her sensitivities to chemicals have become less since she stopped taking all the medications she was offered, but her reactions to many foods have become more pronounced. 'These also still bother me – formaldehyde, reading materials, synthetics and electrical motors.'

Some two years after her illness began, Jan still has neuromuscular complaints, a high heart rate, diarrhoea, and gastrointestinal problems. She and her husband are prepared to wait it out in their mountain cabin in faith and hope for a normal life again.

'There's one thing I wonder about,' Jan said. 'I went to a reunion of our nursing class. Three have multiple sclerosis and one has died. I wonder . . .' – CCC

TERRY – A Long Way To Go

Terry, 23 when he gave this story, grew up in an impoverished area of an Australian city. He was second youngest in a family of eight where food, let alone nourishing food, didn't appear regularly on the table, and where parental supervision scarcely existed.

'I was into everything, drink, drugs, you name it. I abused my body.'

Terry was apprenticed to an electrician. At 18 he had what he thought was a bad case of influenza and didn't recover.

'I didn't know you could feel so bad. Drug trips and hangovers were nothing to this. I thought I was going to die, and I didn't care. I didn't care about anything.'

He recalls his symptoms as being extreme tiredness, weakness of arms and legs and an inability to put thought into action. 'For instance, I'd think I might as well go down to the pub where my mates were, but somehow I couldn't get myself out the gate. It was weird.'

Terry went to two doctors. 'But what's the use? They can't put a bandage on tiredness. Anyway, they said they couldn't find anything wrong with me.' Instead, encouraged by a neighbour, Terry began reading some of the books from her personal library, books on healthy living, diet and overcoming allergies. Through this neighbour he went to stay with a family in the country. Like them, he became a Born Again Christian. 'I saw that what I'd done in my early life – abusing my body – was what had made it possible for the sickness to take hold of me.'

Farm-produced food, organically grown, and the support of a caring family who insisted that he rest, combined to help Terry recover enough to take a paying job as a labourer on another farm. His reading at that stage had not extended to the dangers of agricultural chemicals. The farmer required him to spray a large area of gorse and brush. He was given no protective gear, and the chemical he used for several days was 2,4,5-T. 'I got so ill I thought I was in hell. I wanted to give up, but was afraid to die.' The Christian family again took him in and nursed him into some sort of convalescence.

Five years after his first illness, Terry is still far from well. He has little energy, sweats for no obvious reason, is very thin, has headaches and often doesn't sleep. A skin rash made him go to a

GP who takes his chemical poisoning symptoms seriously and is seeking specialist help to try to remove the toxins from Terry's system.

'Shall I tell you what my dream is? To get better, of course, but to be the founder of a commune where people with this sickness could come and get better. We'd have pure air and soil and grow our own food. Being sick like this has taught me something.' – CCC

TOM – Rest

Tom, an English banker in his 30s, had been unable to work for more than a year when he gave this interview.

'I had always been healthy except for some symptoms of what I now know to be irritable bowel syndrome. Suddenly I had a very severe 'flu-like illness. No matter what I wore, I felt cold, frozen through and through. I became so weak I couldn't climb stairs. Earlier I'd had an accident in Greece, and I'd felt rather shaken even after I was supposedly recovered. There was a lot of pressure at work. I realise now that my system was run down.'

Tom was eager to get back to work as his mind was in 'usual working order'. His limbs and back continued to ache so that walking was an effort. Three months after returning to his bank he suddenly collapsed, with the same symptoms but worse than before.

'A specialist did all the tests and said there was nothing wrong with me. Others I've met with this complaint say they've all been told "There's nothing wrong with you", but we all know there is.

'A psychiatrist gave me some anti-depressants, which helped a little. I sometimes wonder what sort of person wouldn't get depressed when some unknown illness strikes them down and wipes out their career ... I struggled on and on and at last found a neurologist who told me I had the post-viral syndrome, and that I would be better in two years.'

Headaches and weakness continued to afflict him. He had to use taxis to travel even short distances. His sleep patterns, earlier disturbed, became much worse. Sleeplessness merely made him cling limpet-like to the idea of continuing to work.

'Then I had a psychological breakdown. Altogether I've had three major collapses. Fortunately my office is very supportive – they have staff insurancce. The best advice I got then was to rest – rest completely. It's particularly hard for busy, involved people to accept this, but if you don't rest from the beginning of the illness, you will almost certainly exacerbate the symptoms and prolong your incapacity.

'Now, two years after it began, I can walk for as long as half an hour, use the underground, even go to the theatre. I know several people who have become absolutely better within two years. I keep resting, and I'm hopeful.' – CCC

DANIEL – Avoidance of Almost Everything

Daniel, a former scientist, a New Zealander in his early 40s, has been unwell for 18 years, but was able to go on the sickness benefit only five years ago. He is embittered, frustrated and exhausted by his battle to regain his health. During the years, he has read almost everything there is to read on the subject of immune deficiency diseases, seen specialists in several countries, and is now very well-informed.

Both Daniel's daughters are highly allergic, and share his marked sensitivity to moulds, dust and house mites. Their slightly musty all-timber house contains ionisers and air and water purifiers. Daniel also imports an American dust-sealant to seal carpets and bedding against dust mites.

Daniel describes himself as having had allergies since childhood, and suffering acute bowel pains in the 1960s. He believes that a smallpox vaccination prior to overseas travel in 1970 was the trigger for his descent into chronic illhealth.

'I've been constantly sick since then. The 1976 Russian 'flu epidemic really hit me, then I had pleurisy. Then I was prostrate – simply awful. I had depression, swellings of the scalp and face, swollen ankles, tenosynovitis. The fluctuations in my blood sugar were just wild. I discovered I had allergies to almost everything – including most of the vitamin and trace element supplements available in New Zealand. As a result, I spend horrendous amounts importing non-allergenic supplements from the United States.'

Daniel is now a universal reactor and has chronic candidiasis. He can eat only organically-grown vegetables from above ground – leafy vegetables, cauliflower, peas and beans, grains (except wheat). Meats, dairy products, chicken and eggs, fish, tofu and root vegetables all upset him. His limited diet highlights the need for people with CFS to take nutritional supplements tailored to their individual needs. Though the water quality in his town is said to be one of the highest in New Zealand, it must be purified if it is not to upset him. He is fortunate in that his wife's high salary enables the purchase of vital supplements. Many people with CFS are not as fortunate. Sickness and unemployment benefits do not allow for the large expenditure necessary to keep them well enough to stay out of hospital.

BIO-ENERGETIC REGULATORY MEDICINE

The reliability of diagnosis by bio-energetic regulatory (BER) techniques using electroacupuncture according to Voll (EAV) was the subject of a New Zealand Health Department inquiry in 1986. It followed claims by Matthew Tizard MB, ChB, an Auckland general practitioner, that, out of 500 immune dysfunction patients, the illhealth of 131 was attributable to pesticide residues as indicated by EAV diagnosis. Of the 131 cases, Paraquat was involved in 70 cases, 2,4,5-T in 52, Azulox in 4, and Malathion in 5. The inquiry concluded 'that the method is not a reliable diagnostic technique. Claims of agricultural chemical poisoning based upon this technique must be considered invalid.'[1]

Nevertheless, BER is one of the very few medical approaches to CFS with an average-to-good rate of success. The diagnostic technique (EAV) was developed by a German homoeopathic doctor, Reinholdt Voll, in the 1950s. The method uses specialised equipment to evaluate changes in the resistance to the flow of electricity over acupuncture points on fingers and toes. These changes are brought about by putting various substances contained in glass bottles into the circuit. The skilled operator is then able to judge the body's overall vitality, specific organ functioning, the presence of toxic substances and the appropriate corrective treatment. In the case of chemical residues and other toxins, the treatment would be the use of drainage remedies to stimulate their elimination, vitamin C and hyperbaric oxygen therapy.

Though widely used in Europe, the technique is in its infancy elsewhere. The equipment used is not easy to interpret and its diagnostic reliability depends more on the operator's skill than the readings given by the electronic measuring devices. Dr Julian Kenyon of the Centre for the Study of Alternative Therapies in Southampton, England, and Dr Mike Anderson of Queenstown,

New Zealand, are two of many who are working to improve the approach.

Perhaps because of the real difficulties associated with bio-energetic regulatory techniques in their present stage, there are few doctors outside Europe to use them. There are only four medical doctors and a few homoeopaths and naturopaths in New Zealand to do so. All doctors interviewed consider it helps about 80 per cent of cases, with 20 per cent either not being helped or becoming worse.

Two case studies, reported by Dr Tizard to the Health Department in early 1986, are as follows:

Mr W: This man, a 50-year-old fire officer, was involved in an I.C.I. chemical fire in Auckland in December 1984. Since then he has suffered from extreme fatigue, sleep disturbance, occasional bowel upsets, a skin rash on his right foot, profuse sweating and the loss of nearly all his body hair on trunk and limbs.

EAV examination showed grossly abnormal readings characteristic of a toxic over-burdening. A diagnosis of severe Paraquat and 2,4,5-T toxicity was made. In view of the degree of severity and of multiple herbicide toxicity, he was treated with 30gms vitamin C daily, followed by hyperbaric oxygen. After 25 treatments, EAV readings were normal, and the patient was symptom-free with normal energy levels. A marked improvement began from the sixth treatment. One month later he has maintained this state. The explanation for the loss of body hair was the high concentration of Paraquat from the sweat glands, poisoning the hair follicle with consequent hair loss. The excessive sweating represented the body attempting to excrete the Paraquat.

Mr TJ: This previously fit dairy farmer noticed increasing weakness and fatigue over an 18-month period and then developed increasing shortness of breath. Shortly afterwards he was admitted to hospital in acute heart failure and cardiomyopathy was diagnosed. He remained in intractable heart failure with marked enlargement of the heart and severe limitation of all movement. Cardiologists discussed the possibility of cardiac transplantation.

EAV testing found both Paraquat toxicity and a residual Coxsackie virus, both of which were affecting the heart, the most stressed organ. He made a remarkable recovery with homoeopathic Paraquat, being virtually recovered after his sixth treatment. He also received a modified course of Coxsackie virus. He is now able to do a full day's work. X-rays show the heart has returned to normal size.

ECOLOGY CLINICS

Chemical residues are now found in the bodies of almost all Americans with a resulting high incidence of environmentally-caused illness. Ecology and detoxification clinics are springing up in the United States to provide the type of treatment required to return chemical victims to health.

One such clinic is Human Environmental Medicine of San Diego, California, which offers medically managed detoxification programmes against bodily stored environmental contaminants, drugs and alcohol. It uses gas chromatography, mass spectrometry and standard tests to diagnose the presence of toxins. Removal is through a bio-toxic reduction regime of saunas, exercise and nutritional supplementation. The clinic claims that a 70-99 per cent removal of toxins is accomplished within 30 days, with a 70-95 per cent improvement rate in the patients' symptoms.

'Patients will do better to detox than with other methods of therapy. We have had many in three to twelve months who are able to go back into noxious areas and have no effect. Most chemical exposure is reversible, and that is what we bank on,' says Zane Gard MD, the clinic's medical consultant.[2]

Two case studies from the clinic's files illustrate the effects of chemical poisoning, particularly upon the nervous system.[3]

Beth: This 31-year-old chemical victim lived within a mile of a San Diego landfill for 18 years. It is now no longer in use due to suspected public health risks as large amounts of toxic industrial waste were illegally dumped there.

Beth developed asthma when aged eight, following a serious bout with measles. She reported a seven-year history of chronic yeast infections. By the time she was 24 she was disabled due to 'non-specific causes'. Symptoms ranged from dizziness, head pain and pressure, confusion, depression, anxiety states, insomnia, poor memory, lack of concentration, persistent 'flu-like symptoms, fevers, swollen glands, general weakness, numbness of the fingers and facial areas, temporary paralysis of arms upon arising, and a tingling sensation across her scalp.

She was evaluated by 35 doctors in eight years, with no relief of symptoms. She became a candidate for intensive psychotherapy, shock treatment and possible admission to the county mental hospital due to prolonged suicidal states. Upon becoming aware of her immune system dysfunction and chemical intolerances she isolated herself in a chemcially-free bedroom for nine months to allow her immune system to rebuild itself. She experienced immediate relief from symptoms, and left the room only with a portable oxygen apparatus.

Elevated toxin levels were detected by the clinic in a fat biopsy in 1984, and Beth went through the detoxification programme. Her condition has improved by 85 per cent. With a far greater tolerance to chemicals, Beth is no longer confined to a totally controlled environment. Her chronic eye and head pains have disappeared.

Warren: This 38-year-old man has an 11-year history of personality changes, headaches, nausea, cardiac palpitations, joint pains, anxiety, depression, insomnia and memory loss. The onset of these symptoms occurred one year after working as a landscape gardener. He carried a variety of organophosphates and chlorinated hydrocarbons with him inside his truck, using them frequently on his job and later storing them at his home. He did not wear protective clothing or respiratory devices while on the job.

Initial symptoms were headache, nausea and general malaise. Gradually this developed into daily problems with diarrhoea, gas and bloating. Over the next several years his body began to ache with muscle cramping, severe headaches, anxiety, depression, and rapid mood swings. By 1984 he was no longer able to work and was disabled. He completed the BRT programme with a marked improvement of symptoms. When last seen at the clinic, he was free of anxiety, depression and headaches.

Chapter 7   CASE HISTORIES

1   N.Z. Health Department, *Task Force on Chronic Agricultural Chemical Poisoning Notifications: Report to the Director General of Health*, June 1986.

2   'Bioaccumulation of Toxic Chemicals', interview in *Complementary Medicine*, Sept/Oct 1986.

3   Gard, Z.R., 'Bio-Toxic Reduction Program Participants (Condensed) Case Histories', in *Townsend Letter for Doctors*, June 1987, 48.

CANDIDA AND IMMUNE DYSFUNCTION

> Men are naturally most impressed by diseases
> which have obvious manifestations, yet some of
> their worst enemies creep up on them un-
> obtrusively.   RENE DUBOS

Candidiasis, or systemic overgrowth of the yeast candida albicans, is
considered by clinical ecologists and holistic therapists to be the
provocative agent in much chronic and degenerative disease. The
medical establishment may still disagree. Nevertheless, many reputable general practitioners are finding that fungal overgrowth is
increasingly widespread because of the declining vitality of a
growing number of people. Fungal illnesses have become much
more common in recent years and are often complicated by
parasitical infections. These unpleasant manifestations of both the
vegetable and animal world within the body are recognised symptoms of depressed immunity.

Candidiasis is by far the best known of the fungal diseases. In
healthy people, yeasts live harmoniously with other bacteria and
enzymes in the digestive tract. When immune competency declines,
burgeoning candida will further depress the immune system, and
upset the nutrient absorption to such an extent that healing
processes cannot get under way. In the healthy person, with a
healthy immune response, candida creates no problems. In those
who are debilitated and have weakened immunity, as with AIDS
and cancer, this normally mild yeast can turn into an invasive
fungus which infests the esophagus, lungs, stomach, brain, repro-

ductive organs and other tissues and cause many confusing, hard-to-live with symptoms.

Because of diagnostic difficulties, figures on the incidence of yeast-caused disease are difficult to obtain. 'Thrush', a vaginal condition caused by candida albicans, is acknowledged to be very common. A 1979 British dental report estimated that between 29-50 per cent of Britons have oral candida infections. Some claim that yeast-caused problems are epidemic. There is certainly an epidemic of medical literature on candida. Candida albicans is now being implicated in conditions as apparently unrelated as psoriasis, multiple sclerosis, myasthenia gravis, schizophrenia, autism, intractable depression, Crohn's and Meniere's diseases, allergies, systemic lupus erythematosus, tenosynovitis, meningitis and endometriosis. People with endocrine disorders and imbalances are likely to have yeast problems, as are diabetics, whose legs and feet can have particularly high candida levels. Candidiasis is almost guaranteed for heroin addicts, and it is often the first sign of AIDS.

This is no new plague. Hippocrates mentions it circa 400 BC. Candida albicans is just one of the large family of candidas and assorted fungi, all of which live mainly in dark warm body crannies, particularly the digestive tract and reproductive system. Many different factors encourage yeast overload. Modern lifestyles and modern medicine can depress the immune system and feed candida the foods on which it thrives. Particularly implicated are antibiotics, especially the broad spectrum types; diets rich in sugar and yeast; meats with residues of hormones and antibiotics; birth control pills.

The two doctors who have done most to promote awareness of the part that candida plays in ill health are William Crook and Orian Truss, both Americans. Dr Crook says, 'It is important to emphasise that yeast-related health problems are not simply "yeast infections". Instead, they are manifestations of a disorder of the immune system. When the immune system is impaired, yeasts thrive on the mucous membranes, putting out toxins that cause further impairment of normal body function.'

Dr Truss outlines the development of chronic candidiasis in his book, *The Missing Diagnosis*. From being a harmless passenger in the gut, it may make its presence known by symptoms which may be brief, intermittent, chronic or acute. Their effects may be limited to the seat of infection – anywhere in the intestinal tract from mouth to rectum, the skin or nails, or they can affect all parts of the body, including the brain.

Candida albicans is a dimorphic organism which can exist in two forms. The first is a non-invasive sugar-fermenting yeast cell, whereas the fungal state produces long root-like mycelia which can penetrate the intestinal mucosa. This penetration breaks down the barrier between the contents of the intestines and the rest of the body, allowing many incompletely digested dietary proteins to enter the bloodstream. This, and its suppression of suppressor T cells, explains why people with chronic candida overgrowth commonly have many allergies.

The exploding population of yeast spores, living and dying in their billions, affects several functions of the blood. There is depression of B and T cell functioning and blocked lymphocyte responses. A high yeast count will stiffen the red blood cells, making it difficult for the platelets to pass through the capillaries. The blood is thicker and sludgier. The consequent lowered oxygen levels encourage further yeast growth.

Other strategies of this pathogen reported in recent medical literature include widespread depression of enzyme activity. This affects the functioning of many metabolic processes – processes integral to the way the body produces energy from foods, the processing of waste products and healing and body renewal. Disruption of carbohydrate and sugar metabolism can lead to specific intolerances and fluctuating blood sugar levels in the body, with accompanying energy and mood upsets. Disruption of the ammonia cycle means that ammonia is not metabolised properly, with resulting sensitivity to ammonia. Enzyme deficiencies may indeed be the major factor in cot deaths, according to the Sheffield research team studying that problem.

Systemic effects include sore and aching joints, puffy skin and tissues, rashes and inexplicable pains. The female reproductive system can be seriously affected, with ovarian autoimmune damage. Resulting symptoms include the pre-menstrual syndrome, post-natal depression, painful periods, pelvic inflammatory disease and endometriosis. There is also disruption of collagen production and a synergistic relationship with staphylococcus. Staphylococcal infections can be lethal when candida levels are high. Autoimmune symptoms may appear when lowered suppressor T cell activity enables the immune system to attack normal tissues. Autoimmune processes are also set in motion when organs, though not infected by yeast, react allergically to circulating yeast toxins. These include chemicals as unpleasant as acetaldehyde and ethanol. Studies made as far apart as at the New York Hospital-Cornell Medical Centre and at Otago University, New Zealand, found both chemicals in stool samples of people with candidiasis. In the main, however, candida overgrowth damages only the way that the body functions.

Many in the medical establishment still dismiss the theories of Drs Truss and Crook as far-fetched and insufficiently backed by research. But evidence is snowballing to support their claims of immune depression, of autoimmune attacks on the endocrine glands and the production of alcohol and alcohol-related products in the body.

Because yeast in the body is so commonly linked with thrush, candidiasis is often seen as a woman's problem. But babies, boys and men are also affected. Candida has been reported in the lungs and digestive tract of foetuses and is increasingly found in sickly babies as intractable nappy-rash and oral thrush, white spots on the tongue and inside the mouth.

Whereas candida overgrowth in women causes hormone levels to fluctuate wildly with accompanying mood swings, in men it is expressed more as chronic fatigue and sour disposition. There is a constancy of effect in men which gives the impression of normal character and personality. Teenage boys appear depressed or ill-tempered, and lacking in ambition. School work suffers severely as a result of intellectual impairment, lethargy and depression. Because those affected often seem to have particularly weak heads where liquor is concerned, they are inclined to turn to other drugs, marijuana in particular. Candida overgrowth is thought by a number of clinical ecologists to have a bearing on today's sharp increase in violence, teenage suicide and drug use.

Today's sexual mores also encourage the spread of candida. 'Yeast infections aren't seen as sexually transmitted,' explains Max Shepherd, professor of experimental oral biology at the Dunedin Dental School in New Zealand, who has carried out major research on yeast-related problems. 'But there is no doubt that a significant number of men have the same strain of candida in their bodies as exists in their partner's vagina.'

The health of a New Zealand couple with severe CFS symptoms improved markedly during a three-month period without sexual intercourse when home remodelling forced them to share a bedroom with their two children. After they moved back into their own bedroom and resumed sexual relations, their symptoms returned. That they sleep on a waterbed may not have been significant, but some M.E. observers believe that the covering of such beds harbours fungal growth.

When a woman develops thrush and other infections, antibiotics are often prescribed. But these promote additional yeast growth by killing off the beneficial bacteria that help control the yeast. Only narrow spectrum antibiotics should therefore be taken, and then only when really necessary. They won't help thrush, and they won't help colds or 'flu. When antibiotics are used, yoghurt or acidophilus should be taken to promote beneficial bacterial growth.

The overgrowth of candida albicans is related to the pH of the body and the tendency towards alkalinisation may encourage it. It also flourishes in low oxygen situations, so that anything which reduces blood levels of oxygen may cause yeast populations to multiply. Cigarette smokers are more susceptible to fungal infections since smoking depresses oxygen levels in the blood and stomach. Those who breathe shallowly also put themselves at risk.

Because candida is a part of everyone's parasitic and bacterial baggage, candida infestations are extremely difficult to diagnose. Stool cultures cannot always be produced, even from people with known candida problems. Cultures from nose, throat, mouth, gums, tongue, anus, rectum, groin and other warm moist spots appear to be more successful. Nevertheless, all those professionals specialising in immune dysfunction warn that the absence of candida in test results is no proof that it is not present.

Laboratory tests for candida overgrowth are being developed. The ImmunoDiagnostic Laboratories in Oakland, California, have a method for testing measured levels of several antibodies directed against candida. This includes a test for anti-ovarian antibodies.[1] Cross-reactions to both candida and ovary indicate the immune process that damages the ovaries and contributes to problems such as in the case study at the end of this chapter. The MetaMetrix Laboratories in Georgia provide an antibody test – high scores of IgG indicate an active overgrowth of candida, while elevated levels of IgE indicate an allergic reaction to the patient's own candida.[2]

Most doctors diagnose by case history, and response to treatment. Conscientious attention to anti-fungal treatments, diet and hygiene are essential if a chronic sufferer is to return to anything like full health.

People on anti-candida medications should be prepared for the Herxheimer reaction. This is a sudden worsening of symptoms which may occur when the candida organisms start being killed off. The symptoms may occasionally be so distressing that alternative treatments may need to be used.

The importance of a holistic approach to candida is illustrated by the case of an AIDS victim who claimed to have brought his AIDS under control, as reported in a Melbourne newspaper in 1986.[3] Following antibiotic treatment which seemed to make him worse, he went to a naturopath who told him that if he did not clear up his candida overgrowth, he had no hope of controlling his other symptoms.

'The first step in controlling the candida was to starve the yeast colonies of their nutrients,' the young man said. 'For the first two weeks, I followed a diet consisting exclusively of fish, steamed vegetables, boiled brown rice and raw greens. I took two Nizoral tablets a day to chase the yeast out of my body. Note that I was meditating three times a day, and receiving regular massage. I believe I was also helped in my recovery by the patient and constant support of the other members of my household. I also took supplements – vitamins A,B,C,D,E, calcium, zinc, potassium iodide and spirulina. As well, I drank two pints of vegetable juices spread out over the day.'

JUDY'S STORY

Through years of misery, this highly intelligent, career-minded, 35-year-old mother of three went the rounds of the medical profession. No one could find anything wrong with her yet her symptoms were real enough. Against a background of inexplicably low blood pressure and deathly exhaustion, Judy suffered through extremely painful menstrual periods, stomach pains, pre-menstrual syndrome, chronic constipation, intermittent deafness and visual problems, migraines, depression, inexplicable shoulder pains, muscular tiredness and weakness, lung infections, frequent streptococcal throats and sinusitis.

Even her brain and central nervous system seemed to be affected. There were unpredicatable bursts of anger, her head felt strangely clouded and her memory and comprehension were affected.

Judy's face often had a strange grey pallor which alarmed her family and friends. Her eyes might be red-rimmed, sore and itchy. Over 5ft 9inches tall, Judy at her lowest ebb weighed just over 98lbs. She had a good appetite and was not anorexic.

She had intractable vaginal thrush although she had taken an oral contraceptive for only a short time on a prescription basis for endometrial problems. She became severely ill after surgery in 1975 for endometriosis, described by her surgeon as the most severe case he had seen. He removed an ovary.

Judy greatly disliked relying on antibiotics but they were constant in her life because of the fevers and infections that had plagued her from the age of two. Yet the more antibiotics she had, the more infections followed.

By 1985, with three children, Judy's recurring endometriosis, pre-menstrual syndrome and heavy periods swung her doctor to the view that her troubles would be over if her uterus was removed. They would leave her half an ovary.

Three painful infections later, she opened the bathroom cabinet door one day and happened to see her teenage daughter's Nilstat. She started to take it.

'Within a couple of days, the depression in my head lifted. I could think better. I was looking forward to things and I could face life constructively. For the first time in 10 years, I wasn't constipated. The perineal soreness and prickling disappeared. I could suddenly see properly again without prickling feelings or being dazzled.'

Judy also found that her lifelong urge for sweet snacks had left her. 'I used to feel so exhausted. I think my body wanted sweet things, and I used to nibble all day long. I loved sugar – but it never gave me much of a boost.'

Her mood swings and pre-menstrual symptoms were also much improved. 'Sometimes I had felt as though I was two people. I'd felt as though I was being taken over. I didn't feel responsible for the way I talked to people or the selfish ways I reacted or for my violent thoughts. But I wasn't dangerous because I knew when to walk away.'

A year after taking Nilstat, Judy is much better but still not totally well. She is now concentrating on an individualised nutritional programme with supplementation.

Judy is concerned about the health of her 17-year-old daughter who is often tired and has continual benign lumps in her breasts. A number have been removed. Judy's five-year-old son has one complaint after another. She now feels that candida may have been involved in the illhealth of both her parents and her sister.

Candida Checklist
In cases of chronic illhealth where no cause has been found, the checklist of indicators for candida which was developed by the American specialist, Dr William Crook, may be helpful.

It includes:
- Having taken antibiotics for acne, or prolonged and repeated courses of broad spectrum antibiotics.
- Having taken birth control pills or been pregnant.
- Having taken Cortisone, Prednisone, or other corticosteroids.
- Feeling worse on exposure to tobacco smoke, perfumes, diesel fumes and other chemical odours.
- Tiredness and depression.
- Poor memory, feelings of unreality, irritability, inability to concentrate, headaches.
- Numbness, tingling, muscle weakness, lack of coordination.
- Thrush, athlete's foot, 'jock itch' or other fungal infections.
- Prostate problems.
- Food allergies.
- Pains in the joints, recurrent sore throats, coughs.
- Feeling worse on damp days, or in mouldy places.
- Feeling worse after food or drink containing yeast.

Controlling Candida Naturally
Optimal nourishment and close attention to hygiene will reduce the need for medications by ensuring better health.

1. Diet: vegetables, fresh fruits in moderation, fresh meat and fish, eggs, wholegrains, nuts, seeds and oils, natural yoghurt.
AVOID ALL SUGAR, BREAD, YEASTS, MILK AND ALL CHEESES, FRUIT JUICES, BEERS, WINE AND SPIRITS, FOODS CONTAINING VINEGAR, DRIED FRUITS, LEFT-OVERS, COFFEE AND ALL TEAS, MUSHROOMS,

PACKAGED OR PROCESSED FOODS.

2. A rotational and varied diet.

3. A complex individually-prescribed mix of yeast-free vitamins and minerals. Garlic may also help.

4. Cleanse your home thoroughly. Get rid of everything that might be mouldy, damp (pot plants, for instance) or has an upsetting smell. Keep your house dry, warm and well ventilated.

5. Stop smoking or using any other social drugs.

6. Avoid birth control pills and antibiotics (where possible).

7. Exercise strict hygiene, especially of the perineum. After bowel movements, women should wipe from the front to the back to avoid introducing candida to the genital area. Wash the area in tepid rather than hot water after bowel movements.

8. Women should wear sanitary pads rather than use tampons during menstruation.

9. Sexual cleanliness: both partners should bath or shower thoroughly before sex, and wash thoroughly afterwards.

10. Wear cotton underwear, and avoid constricting lower garments, such as tight jeans. It is better to wear loose cotton skirts.

11. **Exercise regularly.**

12. Love, touch, laughter, faith, hope and prayer.

RECOMMENDED READING:

Bodey, G.P. and Fainstein, V., *Candidiasis*. Raven Press, N.Y. 1985 (more for the medical professional).

C. Orian Truss, M.D., *The Missing Diagnosis*, Birmingham, Alabama: C. Orian Truss, 1983.

William G. Crook, M.D., *The Yeast Connection*. Professional Books, 1986.

Leon Chaitow, N.D., D.O., *Candida Albicans*, Thorsons, 1985.

Gerson, Dr Max, *A Cancer Therapy: results of fifty cases*. Totality Books, 1958.

Trowbridge, J.P. and Walker, M., *The Yeast Syndrome: How to Help your Doctor Identify and Treat the Real Cause of your Yeast-Related Illness*. Bantam, 1986.

Chapter 8 CANDIDA

1 Trowbridge, J.P., and Walker, M., *The Yeast Syndrome*, Bantam, 1986, pp.114-16.
2 ibid, pp.120-21.
3 *Melbourne Star*, 24 October 1986.

CASE HISTORY: ALISON

Alison, a 28-year-old wife, mother, and secretary of a New Zealand M.E. support group, has had a lifetime of illhealth, culminating in M.E. After five years of CFS symptoms severe enough to be classified as autoimmune, she feels she has now turned the corner towards health. In combating her CFS symptoms, she is correcting the hidden allergies and candida albicans problems which have plagued her most of her life. Had she not worked with such determination to heal her body, her future would have been bleak.

Alison's medical history and genetic inheritance have many negative aspects. Her mother died of cancer; her father of heart disease; she had grandparents with cancer and heart disease. Goitre, allergies, alcoholism and pre-menstrual syndrome blacken her family medical tree. Her husband also has inherited allergies. Together they have endured severe candida problems. Alison has spent much of her life in the damp coldness of Dunedin; her husband comes from not far distant Tapanui.

Their primary school daughter is sickly and hyperactive. She has a crowded dental arch and has very much the same problems as her mother: candida and mould sensitivity; allergies to egg, corn and dyes, salicylate and amine sensitivities. She has benefited from homoeopathic treatment for residual streptococcal toxins, and was recently diagnosed as asthmatic. She became much better on a strict rotational and anti-candida diet.

Compiling a family medical tree was a useful exercise for Alison, and proved most helpful to her doctors (see diagram). She wrote down the disease processes and reasons for death of every family member as far back as she could go. 'I had to find my own entrance into the disease process, and it was very enlightening to take my

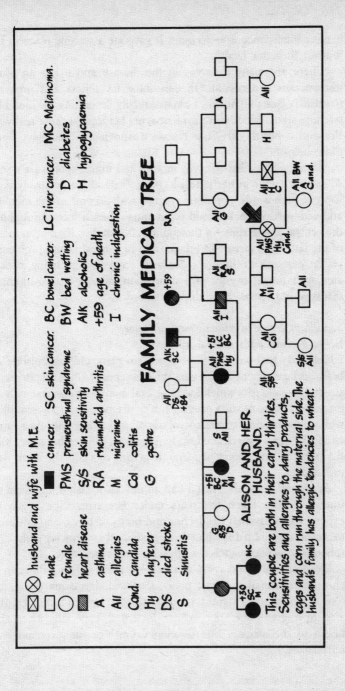

Key:

⊗ husband and wife with M.E.
☒ male
◻ female
▨ heart disease
A asthma
All allergies
Cond. candida
Hy hayfever
DS died stroke
S sinusitis

cancer.   SC skin cancer.   BC bowel cancer.   LC liver cancer.   MC Melanoma.
■ PMS premenstrual syndrome   BW bed wetting   D diabetes
S/s skin sensitivity   Alk alcoholic   H hypoglycaemia
RA rheumatoid arthritis   +59 age of death
M migraine   I chronic indigestion
Col colitis
G goitre

FAMILY MEDICAL TREE

ALISON AND HER HUSBAND.

This couple are both in their early thirties.
Sensitivities and allergies to dairy products,
eggs and corn run through the maternal side. The
husband's family has allergic tendencies to wheat.

genetic inheritance into account. It gave me a starting place in my journey to better health.

'There are many variables in the disease and it has an often idiosyncratic progression. In describing my illness and progress towards reasonable health, I am essentially describing my life. The warning signs, I feel, were evident years before I became really ill. Preventive health care, not rescue treatments, would have been more helpful.'

Alison believes that airborne moulds and fungal spores are a very significant factor in her illhealth. New Zealand has relatively mild winters, high winds, perennial ryegrass with accompanying moulds, and widespread black mould on mountain beech trees throughout the central alpine spine of the country. No studies have been made of the latter two factors in relationship to general health problems, yet factors such as these are generally recognised as being associated with fungal overgrowth, depression, allergies, auto-immune diseases and female reproductive disorders.[1]

Significant events in Alison's medical history:
Birth: Normal with normal infancy.
Childhood: Bed-wetting until about six years old; an episode of boils and persistent skin rash. Wheezy chest. Acute nephritis at six-and-a-half years which led to several months in hospital with an extended course of sulfa drugs. Prior to diagnosis, she was troubled with stomach pains, streptococcal throat, and falling hair. As a small child, she often experienced fits before going to sleep but never told her parents. She always had trouble getting to sleep and often had nightmares.

At around six years, Alison had an unknown rash in the form of watery blisters which left scars under her arms. She began to experience occasional headaches and bouts of hives, and suffered excruciating joint pains which were passed off as 'growing pains'. At school she was considered aggressive and hyperactive.

Her late childhood years were of continual niggling illhealth – chronic constipation, chest pains, sinusitis, dermatitis on hands (one episode) and around nose (persistent). Her headaches graduated to migraine and her weight fluctuated, especially when she began to menstruate. She developed cravings for icecream and milkshakes.

Teenage: There was a period of several months of mild but persistent diarrhoea, vomiting and nausea. For many years she suffered recurrent throat infections; upper respiratory and urinary tract infections; bad ear infections; anaemia and allergic rhinitis. Treatment with sulfa drugs resulted in severe allergic reactions. She began to have typical pre-menstrual syndrome symptoms – mood swings, migraine every few days. These were controlled by oral contraceptives. She was troubled with very dry hair and skin.

Adulthood: Underweight, Alison began to have feelings of unreality. She tired easily and was told to eat more, 'but that made it worse'. Her PMS, urinary tract infections and upper respiratory tract infections were still with her in spite of her continued treatment. All seemed markedly worse in winter.[2] High blood sugar levels became a problem. Migraines became more frequent. Two food allergies were identified – dairy products and wheat. Following two years of thrush, she had ovarian cyst surgery.

1981: Alison's pregnancy was heralded by hives, but otherwise she felt very well and her migraines disappeared. A haemorrhage precipitated a caesarean birth six weeks early. Alison's PMS came back with a vengeance after that. 'I never felt well again,' she said.

1982: Alison was a very exhausted young mother with a difficult, colicky baby. Her own skin and hair became so oily she took to shampooing her hair daily. She had PMS three weeks out of four and felt puffy and uncomfortable for much of the time. She was hospitalised after an anaphylactic reaction to an antibiotic and was found to have low resistance to candida albicans. She became ever more exhausted. Her blood pressure went up to such an extent that she was given diuretics.

1983: During the Tapanui 'flu outbreak, Alison contracted Coxsackie B virus which became persistent, sometimes with dramatic symptoms such as sudden chills and shaking. She found it impossible to sleep well at night and needed afternoon sleeps and quantities of aspirin. Her exhaustion became extreme and her food sensitivities multiplied to the extent that her diet became very limited. She began taking oil of evening primrose which helped the PMS, fluid retention, mood changes and 'spaced-out' feelings.

1984: Alison suffered further deterioration with muscle fatigue, shaking, loss of coordination; pains in shoulders, neck and back; aching limbs; nausea, sweating, hot and cold flushes, light sensitivity; scratchy throat and prickly lung feeling; sneezing, headaches and migraines. Her memory seemed to vanish. Her face was white and waxy, with dark rings round her eyes. Her fingers were numb. She describes herself as jumpy and nervy, crying 'for nothing'. She thought she was dying.

Early in 1984, Alison tried an elimination diet which achieved a dramatic improvement, but which also tipped her into hypersensitivity with nothing much left to eat which didn't make her ill. Salicylates provoked a stupor-like condition in which she was not able to talk or coordinate properly. She went to an allergy clinic where she was treated for multiple allergies (48 food allergens and 4 inhaled allergens). She was sensitive to foods containing salicylates and amines, and petrol fumes, perfumes, formaldehyde and household mould.

An anti-candida regime produced an excellent response. Symptoms which disappeared were: sweating (especially at night), migraine, shaking, nausea, extreme fatigue and aching muscles, slow speech, dizziness, ulcers in the mouth; sensitivity to light, sound, alcohol and touch; headaches; sore throat and sore tongue. Alison's chemical and food allergies were reduced while on the anti-candida treatment.

1985: Alison and her family moved further north. Apart from the incessant nor-west winds, the drier climate suited Alison. Her allergy problems started to decrease. She believed that her troubles might be over, but another virus infection developed into a persistent upper respiratory tract infection. Electroacupuncture was used to diagnose and treat (with injections) a residual streptococcal infection which her new doctor felt dated back to childhood. When the respiratory infection cleared, she was able to stop the allergy injections which had already proved so helpful.

'Though I felt healthier and more energetic, candida was still a bother. I couldn't reduce the Nystatin dosage. If I went off the candida diet, I had sudden bloating, pain, diarrhoea, and headache,' Alison said.

1986: She kept to a strict diet and continued with oil of evening primrose and anti-candida medication. Lactobacillus yoghurt gave her gastritis and arthritis symptoms ('the gut flora must have been wrong'). She began candida immunotherapy and took digestive enzymes for high fat/carbohydrate meals, or when she ate meat more than once a day. No sugar or foods containing yeast and only a little fruit were allowed.

1987: Alison joined a fitness course designed for M.E. sufferers, and found it most helpful. She became much less allergic to the environment. Autoimmune symptoms such as ovarian pain, mid-cycle bleeding and constipation disappeared. She both looked and felt infinitely better. A committed Christian, Alison is also convinced that her healing process was helped by regular prayers offered for her by a group at her church.

Nevertheless Alison and her husband decided to move to Australia, as they had discovered on holidays that the dry climate of Adelaide suited the whole family.

Nine months later, at the time of writing, the health of Alison and that of her husband and daughter is much improved. The asthmatic attacks have almost disappeared. Two months ago, the daughter took herself off Intal voluntarily (sodium cromoglycate). She had previously taken it almost daily for her severe asthma. Her bedwetting stopped shortly after that.

The only major setback experienced by the family was when their household goods arrived from New Zealand. As the cases were opened, out came familiar New Zealand moulds with resulting asthmatic attacks for husband and daughter, and chronic CFS symptoms for Alison.

'I think with the removal of mould stimulus, my system is cleansing itself. I'm rapidly recovering my energy, and have no candida problems at all,' Alison wrote in March 1988.

Comment

Dr Chris Reading, a Sydney genetic counsellor and ortho-molecular psychiatrist, had made an extensive study of autoimmune-disease-prone families, and constructs family medical trees to help track down the basic cause of such tendencies.[3]

Dr Reading links hereditary metabolic weaknesses and hidden allergies with family tendencies to diseases like those in Alison's family. He calls them 'allergy indicators' and he corroborates what CFS specialists are saying: hidden allergies to food and chemicals in food create faulty metabolism and other negative body processes. If these are not corrected, there is the tendency to progress to more devastating diseases or to pass illhealth on to children.

He recommends that people with family histories of the 'allergy indicators' should have their food allergies and vitamin/mineral levels checked and corrected by a doctor competent in this area.

Alison's sensitivity to climate and weather may be due to the over-stimulating effect on her candida of moulds and pollen carried by winds or nurtured in cold damp weather. There is an old Chinese saying: 'The wind penetrates only a predisposed body.' This may explain why women with candida often have symptom flare-ups, from PMS to endometriosis, during periods of high winds and pollen counts. Even being born during the pollen season can predispose an individual to subsequent hayfever.

Chapter 9   ALISON

1   Trowbridge, J.P. and Walker, M., *The Yeast Syndrome*, Bantam Books, 1986, reports on environmental moulds, p.282.
2   Dr Bill Rea, speaking at the 1983 Yeast-Human Interaction Symposium, San Francisco, described the incidence of female reproductive problems increasing markedly at times of high mould and pollen counts in a controlled survey in Texas.
3   Reading, C. and Meillon, R., *Relatively Speaking – The Family Tree Way to Better Health*, Fontana, 1984. Dr Chris Reading, a Sydney orthomolecular physician, genetic counsellor and psychiatrist, concentrates on inherited vitamin and mineral deficiencies and allergies as risk factors in serious disease.

CASE HISTORY: GERMAINE

Tiny, emaciated 40-year-old Germaine . . . at the peak of her battle with chronic herpesviruses she looked as if she had AIDS. At times she was very close to death. Her apparent inner strength, her acceptance of her illness, her ability to rally when visitors called and her Christian faith held her together through a nightmare 18 years.

Germaine's history of chronic illhealth shows how intractable, confusing and devastating are the symptoms arising from a dysfunctioning immune response. Her history illustrates the cyclical nature of immune-related diseases, with periods of remission, the relapses – and possible recovery. The periods of remission and recovery signify that the immune system temporarily has the upper hand over the persistent pathogens and faulty body functioning.

Germaine's story, she has come to believe, also gives insights into the power of the subconscious, both in its ability to paralyse the immune response, and in activating it. The relationship between mind and body, and how they can work together to promote healing, is now recognised as crucial to the outcome of immune-related disease although each case of course is different.

Before her illness, Germaine was a high achiever, always under pressure, always in a hurry. A New Zealand primary school teacher, she was on several national educational committees which involved frequent air travel to conferences. It is only recently that she has realised how much her stresses affected her interaction with her immediate environment. She now admits to a lifelong inability to remember faces and surroundings. She had a tendency to gulp her food, thereby taxing her digestion, and giving her salivary enzymes little chance to assist with digestion.

In 1970, most of the children at Germaine's school caught

chickenpox. She followed with a painful rash around her waist. It was first thought to be a streptococcal infection; then herpes zoster (shingles). It blistered and spread. She woke one morning without the use of her legs. During a month in hospital, Germaine was given a painful myelogram (X-ray of the spinal cord) which showed nothing. She was discharged little better than when she went in and her case was regarded as a medical mystery. She was given a year's sick leave on full pay.

During the next 10 years some remissions followed, but were overshadowed by long episodes of extreme muscle weakness, back problems, general exhaustion and other symptoms. By 1980 Germaine was a total invalid, often helpless, incontinent, unable to feed or bath herself. Her muscles were so weak that even knitting was impossible, and a bone snapped in her hand when she lifted a kettle. Her teeth changed colour and looked grey and opaque. Her eyelid muscles were so weak that keeping her eyes open was sometimes difficult. A multiple sclerosis support group could give her little help as her symptoms were not typical.

Persistent sleep disturbance plagued her – an hour or two initial sleep after going to bed, then wakeful, restless nights. During the day Germaine would doze intermittently. She took sleeping tablets for 17 years, except during crisis times when they made her feel too ill. Urinary frequency and flatulence added to her miseries. Although she was as thin as a concentration camp survivor, her stomach always protruded like a ball. After her scanty meals her mother would help her bring up wind, patting her back as if she were a baby. On one occasion they counted more than 200 belches.

Germaine developed multiple allergies during her illness. She reacted particularly to all flavourings and preservatives, to all milk products, to gluten, to monosodium glutamate, to wheat, to salicylates (found in peas and most fruits), to some vegetables, to nitrates and amines. The smell of printer's ink made her ill so that she couldn't read a newspaper.

She was frequently told by medical specialists that her problems 'could be psychological', that she needed a man, that she wanted to gain her mother's attention, that she was jealous of her twin sister. Both she and her own doctor resented these statements.

Germaine's vital forces have at times drained to almost nothing. Her GP told her in late-1986 that she must conserve her energies to provide strength for her vital organs. At that time her life was in doubt.

Medical notes:

The younger of twins, with a normal birth. Developed early allergies to berry fruits and new season apples (salicylates). Her lymph glands were swollen for several years. As a teenager she had severe sinusitis. Her livelier twin sister had similar allergies and sinusitis, but no immune problems developed in later life.

1969: Germaine suffered from severe diarrhoea for 6 months following her twin sister's marriage. Bowel X-rays were negative. It was later confirmed that apples caused the diarrhoea.

1970: Herpes zoster (shingles), hospitalisation and year's sick leave. She worked through 1971-75, never well, but managing to get through the day.

1975: Digestive upsets, migraine, muscle and joint pains. Blood tests and X-rays showed nothing. Germaine nevertheless improved sufficiently to take an overseas trip to further her studies in primary education. Following pre-trip immunisations she spent a week in bed. She became severely ill overseas, collapsing in the U.S.A. Tests showed nothing (except pregnancy – and Germaine wasn't pregnant). She was given cortisone injections for fibrositis, and ultrasonic massage for pain and muscle tension. Those gave her no relief and she had to rest 3 months before returning home.

1976: Though in constant severe pain, Germaine went back to teaching from 1976-80. She had regular hydrotherapy treatment for pain relief which provided no lasting help. She turned to alternative therapies in 1977 but after 3 months' acupuncture she was no better. She then had 6 months of twice-weekly visits to a chiropractor. This only made her worse.

Germaine had constant colds and influenza during the next four years, for which she received antibiotics. She became allergic to antibiotics, anti-inflammatory drugs, Disprin and a wide range of foods. Her coordination became poor, she tripped, fell and dropped things constantly. She was weak and tired, her memory failed her. She cut down on many activities.

1978: Following 2 weeks' sick leave for rest and the treatment of exhaustion, she visited a colour therapist who told her that her body lacked calcium and was full of toxins. (She now believes this to be correct.) She took a course of vitamins and ascorbic acid, and avoided wheat and sugar. After six months, she was no better. She had a hospital consultation in which she was interviewed by seven people at once. They told her nothing was organically wrong and recommended psychiatry. Her GP was horrified, and did not follow up the recommendation.

1980: Germaine resigned from teaching because of ill health. Blood tests showed abnormal immunoglobulin levels. She received vitamin B12 injections weekly for 6 months with no relief; also magnesium for indigestion, pain killers and sleeping drugs. Her diet was still conventional, though 'no junk food'.

1981: Blood tests were slightly positive for arthritis.

1982: Germaine consulted Dr Hawe, a Sydney rheumatologist, who diagnosed clear-cut symptoms of M.E. A muscle biopsy showed no specific abnormalities. She was referred to immunologist Dr Robert Loblay of Sydney Univesity for seven months' allergy testing through an exclusion diet. This was before the importance of rotational eating was realised. For seven months she ate nothing but potatoes, lettuce, parsley, chicken, lamb, beef, rice and pears. No sauces, gravies, butter or milk. Everything was steamed, boiled or microwaved. Some symptoms subsided, particularly the pain and digestive upsets, but she became weaker.

1982-86: Her debility increased. She spent each winter in bed. Mestinon was prescribed to stimulate her muscles, with no improvement. Severe side effects included muscle and throat spasms (when eating).

1984: Started a rotational, anti-fungal diet with no sugar, little carbohydrate. She started on Nystatin but there was no marked improvement.

1985: Consulted Dr X, a GP specialising in bio-regulatory medicine, using a Vega machine for EAV readings. These confirmed persistent herpes zoster virus and streptococcal residues. Dr X gave her a course of 10 homoeopathic injections to drain her body of toxins but paid no attention to diet, apart from avoidance of the foods to which she was sensitive. Germaine was much improved at the end of the eight month course of treatment.

1986: She relapsed completely in May (the beginning of the Southern hemisphere winter). EAV readings showed herpes zoster still present. Another course of 10 injections was started. There was some improvement when re-tested in September. She then became extremely weak and unable to tolerate even the smallest amounts of formerly acceptable foods. She weighed only 84lbs and death seemed imminent. Her specialist GP appeared uninterested and her GP agreed she should have a second opinion from Dr Y, a well-qualified general practitioner and acupuncturist specialising in bio-regulatory medicine.

Dr Y felt that candida, shingles and a streptococcal infection were only symptoms of far more deep-seated problems which went back to Germaine's childhood allergies. He believed that her immune system was almost non-functioning. Pulses at different acupuncture points showed profound bodily weakness and acute malnutrition. Dr Y started her on a course of Parenterovite vitamin and mineral injections, vitamin B12 and Iscador injections. After a day's fasting and a day of raw vegetable juice, Germaine went on an all-leaf vegetable diet (the first week, blended; the second week, steamed). She also took homoeopathic candida drops.

1987: Her biggest physical setback during the months in which she slowly regained her health was a two-month period of agonising back pains. Dr Y treated the pain with simple electro-magnetic therapy – a small pad giving off a low electrical field on her back, and small therapeutic magnets taped to other sore spots. In late 1987 Germaine found that wearing small magnetic bracelets improved her circulation and colouring and gave her whole nights of good sleep. Their benefit was, however, only temporary.

1988: Germaine is now going for short walks, doing a little shopping, driving her car, going to the library, reading, teaching Sunday School, and working on a recipe book for people with allergies. She has put on 20lbs, grown half-an-inch, and her teeth are white again.

Like many of the more desperate (and less conventional) people with allergies, Germaine began using a pendulum as an aid to detecting foods, drugs and chemicals to which she was intolerant, and in assessing suitable levels of nutritional supplements and medication. Her experiences are recounted in Chapter 14, *Self Help*.

She has begun a course of Enzyme Potentiated Desensitisation, to which her initial reactions were severe although she is now responding well.

She now sees significance in the vivid dreams that occurred regularly throughout her illness. (Unlike some chronic fatigue syndrome patients, Germaine had no delusions or hallucinations.) In her dreams, she was often lost in terrifying mazes, or unable to find her way out of large dark houses.

Coming to grips with improved health after so many years of being ill has been very difficult for her, she says. She is finding that regular art therapy with a Steiner-trained therapist is unlocking emotions she didn't know she had.

Germaine says she is willing to change and grow and explore every possible avenue, but her search for health is not over. Medical tests and investigations continue.

BRAIN AND BODY

The individual self is like a passenger in the chariot of the material body, with intelligence as the driver. The mind is the driving instrument, and the five senses are like the pulling horses. Thus, the self is the enjoyer – or sufferer – in the association of the mind and senses.   BHAGAVAD GITA, *Ch. 6, v. 34.*

Even the dreariest of clouds must have its silver lining. The chronic fatigue syndrome with its extraordinary fatigue, depression and pernicious symptomology is forcing Western medicine to recognise the links between brain and body and the uniqueness of every single patient. Each individual with the syndrome can be understood only in terms of that particular individual. Each individual's chronic illhealth can be understood only as a facet of that person. It is as though, in an increasingly impersonal and mechanistic environment, sufferers are saying: 'These reactions are *mine alone*; the treatment I must have is special to *me* only. I cannot be fobbed off with mass medications and 10-minute consultations.'

There is now increasing awareness that referring CFS patients to psychiatrists unaware of the importance of brain/body links is likely to be a waste of time and money. Similarly, concentrating on physical symptoms, to the exclusion of all else, can also be eventually self-defeating. The awareness is well overdue. The reactions of doctors for centuries to people suffering from illnesses which link body and mind has been to brand them as mentally unstable. The royal physician to King George III, for instance, used confinement, strait-jackets and whipping to treat the King's porphyria, a painful enzyme-related disease with similarities to CFS.[1]

It cannot be stressed too often that the chronic fatigue syndrome is a physical illness. Because CFS strikes such a broad cross-section, however, some people – the usual proportion in the community – will be suffering from emotional disorders when they become ill with CFS. Obviously they will benefit from the right kind of psychological counselling, just as they would have benefited if they had not been stricken with CFS. With this syndrome every circumstance must be taken into account in the search for health.

The initial outbreaks of CFS, such as that of myalgic encephalomyelitis at London's Royal Free Hospital in 1955, were dismissed as hysteria and anxiety. Those affected were seen as a bunch of neurotics. This attitude has pervaded the medical profession since then. But those who have been unwell for any length of time are not unnaturally anxious. Their terror of illness without end, of perhaps forfeiting the love of those most dear to them and the respect of their colleagues, of failing their friends and themselves, of losing their very reason for living are all fomented by their helplessness in an implacable pattern of relapses and remission. Most feel certain that their feelings of wretchedness do not constitute 'ordinary depression' but are the direct result of their physical illness.

They often have dramatic descriptions of how they feel. 'It is hard to describe the depth of the depression,' said Patrick, a New Zealand university lecturer. 'Sometimes I would wake up with the feeling that my brain was dying. There would be this overwhelming sensation of approaching doom and death, a feeling of utter blackness and disaster as though I – and the world – were coming to an end together.'

Other mental symptoms are of a type which most people experience from time to time, some more frequently than others. To sufferers, their continued presence means endless confusion of thought, perception and speech. 'Scrambled egg brain' or 'a head full of cottonwool' are commonly described, as is the muddling and forgetting of words. 'I put words in the wrong order . . . I muddle two favourite words "nice" and "neat" to produce "neece". I get letters mixed and live in mortal terror of saying a naughty word by mistake,' writes Sylvia, who is struggling through tertiary studies.

The Dean of Westminster Abbey, the Very Rev. Michael Mayne,

writes of his experiences with the syndrome in his book, *A Year Lost and Found*. Of his mental symptoms he says: 'It was as if my brain had seized up, and I would find myself groping for familiar words, and failing to listen or take in what I was told. I was both aware and unaware of this: too withdrawn into myself and too emotionally diminished to do much about it.'[2]

More severe mental disturbances may be experienced from time to time, along with the usual physical symptoms. Particularly vivid dreams, sometimes turning into horrifying nightmares, are frequently reported, as are hallucinations just before going to sleep. Alison (Chapter 9) had childhood bedtimes haunted by frequent and frightening hallucinations and seizures. Psychotherapists explain these as 'unresolved issues of the psyche'. Clinical ecologists recommend that the possibility of biotin deficiency should be examined.

Dr Peter Behan of the Glasgow Institute of Neurological Sciences, and Ayrshire GP, Dr K.G. Fegan, noted 'brainstem signs' in all M.E. patients studied. They reported symptoms (which are also associated with the cerebral cortex and limbic system) such as: lack of concentration, loss of memory, depression and anxiety without an apparent cause, drowsiness, lethargy, tinnitus, extended periods of sleep, hallucinations at the beginning of sleep, and giddiness.[3]

Celia Wookey, a British general practitioner and M.E. sufferer, describes brain symptoms in her book *Myalgic Encephalomyelitis*. 'I have seen cases of M.E. present as a personality disorder in which irritability (characteristically worse before meals) and delusions of persecution may be the predominant features.'[4] Surrey therapist Tuula Taormaa finds that many of her CFS patients suffer from agoraphobia, anxiety and panic attacks. She has found that the correction of any underlying hypoglycaemia is usually helpful.

Harold N. Levinson MD, a Canadian physician, says that anxiety disorders, phobias and fears may also be associated with cerebellar-vestibular (CV) dysfunction. (Movement and balance are both determined by the cerebellum and the vestibule of the ear.) In various studies of 20,000 CV dysfunctioning individuals, 90 per cent had fears, phobias and panic attacks. These were found to be related to their CV dysfunction by the most sophisticated of tests. The onset of phobic symptoms usually followed something that upset CV function: stress, toxins, infections, viruses and degenerative disorders.

'Many CEBV patients have vestibular disorders,' Gidget Faubion, national president of the U.S. Epstein-Barr Virus Association, said.[5] 'My original diagnosis was tentative MS because I kept falling over coffee tables and things. I weighed 85 pounds – that's typical of CV patients. They are misdiagnosed, mishandled, mistreated, given the wrong kind of drugs, given the wrong kind of therapy, and they go through years and years of this before being properly diagnosed.'

Cerebellar-vestibular symptoms include fear of heights and falling, fears of driving or swimming, 'jelly legs', fears of lifts and elevators, trains, planes and buses, getting easily lost, claustrophobia, panic attacks and obsessive behaviour.[6]

Candida overgrowth as a major factor in depression, irritability, feelings of unreality and inability to think properly (all of which are very much involved in CFS) is, as yet, recognised by only a few medical professionals though well documented in clinical ecology journals and in the popular press. Candidiasis and candida sensitivity have also been suggested as an underlying factor in psychotic illness. Two such cases clearly involved candida:[7]

• An English woman whose life was scarred by violent schizophrenic or manic-depressive breakdowns, periods of intractable depression and fluctuating mystery pains in her stomach (which were soothed only by milk), finally became intolerant to many foods. Consultation with a clinical ecologist revealed she was a multiple reactor with candida overgrowth. Attention to diet and candida removal resulted in the end of her pains and the emergence of her normally cheerful, strong nature. She now finds she is highly sensitive to all chemicals and has adapted her home environment accordingly.

• A New Zealand farming woman who spent nine years as a manic-depressive in a mental institution told of her conviction throughout those years that she was not mad, but that something terribly wrong was going on in her body. 'I used to look around the ward at the other women, and think "Poor things, they are just like me, and no one is bothering to find out what is wrong".' This woman's family read about candida and allergies, had her released from hospital and treated by a sympathetic and open-minded GP. Her brain symptoms have now cleared to the point where she is leading a normal life. She is, however, particularly sensitive to agricultural chemicals.

Candida specialist Orian Truss MD lists some of the candida-caused mechanisms affecting brain functioning: metabolic disturbances in neurons, membrane abnormalities, impairment of acetylcholine synthesis, defective neurotransmitter functioning, and diminished oxygen delivery.[8] Brain symptoms are also associated with allergies which can swell brain tissues or introduce foreign proteins into the brain. Just as with candida overgrowth, allergies and chemicals can disrupt hormone and enzyme pathways connecting brain and body.

Most pesticides are designed to destroy nerve functioning in insects and small rodents. Since human nervous systems are not so different, concern is growing about the neurotoxic effect of pesticides on human nerve functioning. Depending on individual body burdens of chemicals and individual immune strength, enzyme functioning and hormonal pathways may be damaged. The resulting neurotoxic effects run the gamut from subtle changes in brain waves and behaviour to drowsiness, irritability, severe mental deterioration, uncontrollable shaking and crippling nerve damage.

Particular concern is directed at pesticide effects on acetylcholine processes integral to many body functions. B.B. Young describes what happens in *Journal of Pesticide Reform*: 'All operate by intensifying the effects of acetylcholine, a chemical that serves as a courier to relay impulses from one particular type of nerve cell to the next. Under ordinary circumstances, after the second nerve cell has received the incoming pulse, the acetylcholine courier is taken out of action by an enzyme called acetylcholinesterase (commonly referred to as cholinesterase). The pesticides interfere with this step by binding to and monopolising the enzyme, so that the now-unattended acetylcholine continues to deliver its stimular signals without allowing any time for the nerve to rest.'[9]

Elevated acetylcholine activity in the brain can produce headache, lethargy, inability to concentrate and disorientation. Even after cholinesterase activity returns to normal (as it does usually within hours, although it can sometimes be weeks or months), other enzymes continue to be affected. Victims notice sensations of pain, and tingling and numbness in their legs and feet followed by increasing weakness and clumsiness which make it difficult to walk or to handle objects.

Pesticides (particularly the organophosphates and carbamates) thus can have subtle and delayed effects on brain function: persistent mental and behavioural problems, drowsiness, speech defects, poor concentration, memory lapses and emotional instability.[10] Toxic chemicals specialist Dr Douglas Seba questions basic assumptions about food intolerances when he says: 'Doesn't this all sound so familiar? Doesn't it sound like allergies?'

The brain's interaction with the immune system was discussed in Chapter 5. Numerous studies have shown that allergic reactions occurred when people believed they were eating or had come in contact with substances normally causing reactions, even when the substance in question was non-reactive. Or conversely, people exposed to highly allergenic substances did not react when they believed the substance to be one which did not harm them. Hypnosis is particularly successful in controlling skin reactions in Type 1 allergies.[11]

It is a matter for debate why some are able to control reactions and not others. American neurologist George Beard, writing more than 100 years ago, may have had the answer. He described the effects of stress on people who 'without being sick . . . with acute disorder, yet are very poor in nerve force. If from overtoil, sorrow or injury, they overdraw their little surplus, they may find that it will require months to make up the deficiency.'[12]

The pattern of illhealth characteristic of the chronic fatigue syndrome bears out the theories of Canadian physiologist Professor Hans Selye. This eminent researcher found that stress affects vulnerability to disease by reducing the efficiency of the immune response. He defined 'stress' in the broadest possible sense – anything that is uncomfortable to mind and body and which affects its smooth running: disease, malnutrition, boredom, helplessness, chemicals in the atmosphere, injury, emotions like lack of self-esteem, fear and anger. Too little activity is as harmful as too much, so that people who have nothing to do are as endangered as those who are overburdened.

In Selye's concept of the General Adaptation Response, GAS, the body switches on all its responses at the first stage of stimulation. If the stress continues for some time, the body becomes used to it, and enters a Stage of Adaptation or Resistance. At this stage, great quantities of corticosteroid hormones are produced in the adrenal glands. This is the stage at which food and chemical intolerances surface. But there is a limit to what the body can bear if the stress goes on too long, and the Stage of Exhaustion sets in. This is when the adrenal glands become exhausted, the other endocrine glands are overtaxed, and there is severe deterioration of physiological functioning and immune strength.

PROLONGED STRESS – some effects on the body

Increases sugar and insulin in the bloodstream . . . hypoglycaemia or possibly diabetes

Increases cholesterol in the blood . . . atherosclerosis and high blood pressure

Thickens the blood . . . less oxygen carried, brain symptoms, strokes, tachycardia

Increases thyroid production . . . nerves, insomnia, weight loss

Increases endorphin release . . . aggravates migraines, backaches and body pain

Increases histamine release . . . allergic reactions

Stimulates harmful levels of cortisone . . . adrenal and lymph glands shrivel, the immune response weakens, stomach ulcers, colitis, brittle bones

Increases breathing . . . hyperventilation and vertigo

Reduces digestive efficiency . . . bloating, diarrhoea, stomach pains

Increases skin pallor . . . skin becomes coarser; hair becomes lifeless and stringy

---

Signs of a brain/body breakthrough are beginning to appear in medical journals. 'Myalgic Encephalomyelitis Presenting as Psychiatric Illness' is the title of a paper in the *British Journal of Clinical and Social Psychiatry* in 1986. It describes how M.E. sufferers may be misdiagnosed and mistreated if their symptoms are thought to be mental. By Adrian Winbow, consultant psychiatrist at Runwell Hospital in Essex, it examines three patients diagnosed as having endogenous depression or phobic anxiety states for whom conventional drug treatment was useless. Following the discovery of immune complexes and viral antibodies, they were diagnosed as having M.E., rested and given appropriate treatment. Their mental state improved along with their energy levels. 'It is obviously important to make an accurate diagnosis in this group of patients, as complete rest from the onset of the illness improves the prognosis considerably,' Dr Winbow comments.[13]

Preliminary information in the ANZMES (N.Z.) journal, *Meeting-Place* July 1988, suggests that some tricyclic anti-depressants, originally developed as anti-histamines, are of value in treating CFS symptoms. 'Antidepressants' are chemicals, and, like any other chemicals, are capable of altering the body's biochemical balance. They do not necessarily act on the mind at all.

Commenting on the very considerable improvements noted by the (as yet small) sample of sufferers taking the tricyclic Prothiaden, *Meeting-Place* suggests that the improvement in mood may be 'because some underlying biochemical process has been partly corrected'. (That 'partly' is a reminder that all health-promoting factors must be taken into account, and that no single treatment or approach is sufficient with chronic fatigue and immune dysfunction.)

What else of the future? A review paper, 'Postviral fatigue syndrome: time for a new approach', appeared in the *British Medical Journal* in March 1988.[14] In it Dr Anthony David of London's Maudsley Psychiatric Hospital and his colleagues say they believe that 'the complex and rapidly developing science of psychoneuroimmunology may yet shed light on our understanding of the postviral fatigue syndrome'. This science, so new that it goes under a variety of names, including psychosomatic medicine, psychoimmunology and neuroimmune-modulation, is being developed by an alliance of psychiatrists, immunologists, neuroscientists and microbiologists who are looking beyond the confines of their own disciplines. They agree that the subconscious mind must always be respected, since it can sabotage the most sincere efforts people make to heal themselves.

William Collinge, counsellor and behavioural therapist at Incline Village, Nevada, has worked with literally hundreds of immune dysfunction patients. 'The way to work with the subconscious in healing is first to discover what are the deeper attitudes towards the illness. Then you can explore to what degree those attitudes are serving the patient, and suggest that they can be changed. Since the subconscious is directly linked to the physical body, it is intimately involved in influencing bodily states, including immune functioning. The subconscious can be a great friend and ally in fighting disease, if the patient can make friends with it and present a united front.'

Psychoneuroimmunology is based on the premise that the brain is one with the body and that hormones come together to do the brain's bidding. It envisions hormone and enzyme systems with links to everything else, and molecular messengers ferrying information between brain, immune system and the body. This oneness of mind and body is demonstrated as researchers find that hormones thought once to be manufactured solely in the brain are manufactured in lungs, gut and endocrine glands, and that hormones formerly thought to be manufactured elsewhere in the body are also manufactured in the brain (see diagram). Harvard neurosurgeon Richard Bergland stresses that if humanity is to benefit from this new knowledge, whole new strategies of education must be developed for those who provide health care. He predicts that physicians and scientists will measure brain hormones, will link them to specific diseases, and will devise 'space-age techniques to restock the mind's hormonal pantries'. Molecules, more than mind-altering drugs, will be crucial in restoring the health of the previously incurable.[15]

Selected Hormones and Sites of Production throughout the body

HORMONE NAME	OTHER ORGAN SITES				
	Brain	Pituitary	Adrenal	Gut	Gonads
Acetylcholine	✕	✕	✕	✕	✕
Adrenalin	✕	✕	✕	✕	✕
Serotonin	✕	✕	✕	✕	✕
Endorphins	✕	✕	✕	✕	✕
Histamine	✕	✕	✕	✕	✕
Glutamate	✕	✕	✕	✕	✕
Glycine	✕	✕	✕	✕	✕

No patient has been more instrumental in focussing attention on psychoneuroimmunology than the American editor, and now professor of medicine, Norman Cousins. In his book, *Anatomy of an Illness*, he describes the healing power of laughter and the positive emotions of hope, faith and enjoyment during his recovery from a near-fatal connective tissue disease. His blood sedimentation problems and pains in joints and bones gradually faded away on a self-prescribed programme (in partnership with his doctor) which included ascorbic acid and *Candid Camera* and Marx Brothers comic movies. He argues that 'hormones of happiness' exist and are triggered by joy and laughter. 'Both on the conscious and subconscious level, the mind can order the body to react or respond in different ways. Such response involves body chemistry and not just psychological reactions,' he wrote.[16]

Positive thinking, of course, cannot by any means always be successful, but negative thinking never is. In conclusion, these approaches emerge in the treatment of the chronic fatigue syndrome:
● Determined efforts should be made to discover physiological causes for mental symptoms.
● Tricyclic anti-depressants appear to be useful in treating physical symptoms; therapies to eliminate the causes of physical illhealth are helpful for brain symptoms.
● The right kind of psychotherapeutic intervention can often be extremely helpful.
Thus these strategies, along with anti-candida therapy, allergy treatment, the removal of toxins, the normalisation of blood sugar levels, attention to diet, rest, correction of environment and restoration of the body's energies are all important in returning brain and body to full, functional health.

Questions for Looking Within
The following questions may help some people in exploring sub-conscious attitudes about illness. Take time to read each question, close your eyes, and see what answers come. Then write them down. (Reprinted with the permission of William Collinge, Sierra Institute, P.O. Box 3792, Incline Village, Nevada 89450, U.S.A.)

1. Describe your main symptoms.
2. What events do these symptoms remind you of from your past?
3. What emotional events occurred shortly before this illness?
4. What emotion does having this illness make you feel?
5. To what degree have you avoided this emotion in the past?
6. What does this illness keep you from doing?
7. To what degree do you welcome being unable to do these things?
8. Who else is affected by your illness, and how?
9. What are you getting from other people now, that you did not get before having this illness?
10. What life lesson(s) does this illness draw to your attention?
11. In what way might a *part* of you prefer to remain ill?
12. How will your life be different when you are well?

RECOMMENDED READING

The Fabric of Mind, by Richard Bergland, Penguin Books, 1985. An exploration of the brain as a gland, and the way that brain hormones manufactured outside the brain affect behaviour.

Anatomy of an Illness as Perceived by the Patient: reflections on healing and regeneration, by Norman Cousins, Bantam Books, 1981. The record of a successful fight against a frequently fatal disease.

The Joy of Stress, by Dr Peter Hanson. Describes the mechanisms of stress and how they affect the body, and suggests ways of harnessing stress productively. Pan Books, 1987.

The Stress of Life, by Hans Selye, McGraw-Hill, 1978. The most important of all books on stress; suitable for health professionals and informed lay readers.

Brain Allergies: the psycho-nutrient connection, by Wm H. Philpott and Dwight K. Kalita, Keats Publishing Inc, U.S. 1980. A vital resource for the health professional and informed lay person.

Diet, Crime and Delinquency, by Alexander Schauss, Parker House, Berkeley, U.S. Demonstrates how food allergies, junk foods and lead poisoning can foster violence. Brief studies. Good bibliography.

Food, Mind and Mood, by David Sheinkin, Michael Schackter and Richard Hutton, Warner Books, U.S., 1979. Highlights the concepts of energy flow as related to brain sensitivities and testing.

Chapter 11 BRAIN AND BODY

1 Dean, G., *The Porphyrias: a story of inheritance and environment,* Pitman Medical, 1971. Discusses neurosis, hysteria, psychosis and emotional fragility alongside physical symptoms.

2 Mayne, Michael, *A Year Lost and Found,* Darton, Longman & Todd, London, 1987.

3 Fegan, K.G., Behan, P.O. and Bell, E.J., 'Myalgic encephalomyelitis – report of an epidemic', *Jnl. Royal Coll. Gen. Practitioners,* June 1983, Vol 33, No. 251, 335-7.

4 Wookey, C., *Myalgic Encephalomyelitis – Post-Viral Fatigue Syndrome and How to Cope With It,* Croom Helm, 1986, p.38.

5 Personal communication to the author.

6 Watson, M.A. and Sinclair, H., *Balancing Act: for people with dizziness and balance disorders,* Good Samaritan Hospital and Medical Center, Portland, Oregon, 1986.

7 Cases personally observed by the author.

8 Truss, C. Orian, 'Metabolic Abnormalities in Patients with Chronic Candidiasis', *Jnl. Orthomolecular Psychiatry,* 1983, 13:2, 66-93.

9 Young, B.B., 'Neurotoxicity of Pesticides', *Jnl. Pesticide Reform,* Vol. 6, 2, 8-11, Summer 1986.

10 Wagner, S.L., 'Organophosphates', *Clinical toxicology of agricultural chemicals,* Noyes Data Corp., 1983, pp. 205-46.

11 Barber, T.X., 'Changing "Unchangeable" Bodily Processes by (Hypnotic) Suggestions: A New Look at Hypnosis, Cognitions, Imagining, and the Mind-Body Problem', in A.A. Sheikh (ed.) *Imagination and Healing,* Baywood Pub. Co., N.Y., 1984.

12 As reported in: 'An outbreak of encephalomyelitis in the Royal Free Hospital Group, London, in 1955', in *Br. Med. Jnl, 1957; ii:1436-7.*

13 Winbow, A., 'Myalgic Encephalomyelitis presenting as psychiatric illness', in *Br. Jnl Clinical and Social Psychology,* Vol 4 (12986), 2, 30-31.

14 David, A.S., Wessely, S., and Pelosi, A.J., 'Postviral fatigue syndrome; time for a new approach', in *Br. Med. Jnl,* 5 March 1988, 296: 696-9.

15 Bergland, R., *The Fabric of Mind,* Penguin, 1985. Gives a remarkable overview of developing theories relating to brain function, and explains recent research.

16 Cousins, N., *Anatomy of an Illness,* Bantam Books, 1981, p.87.

PART II
Pathway to Health

THE HEALING JOURNEY

> Medical treatment should seek not just to repair damage and restore vital balances but to enhance the quality of life and to help the patient overcome feelings of hopelessness and helplessness. If the physician is to be fully effective in these directions, the patient must be a responsive and appreciative partner.
>
> NORMAN COUSINS, *The Healing Heart*, 1983.

Every person is an individual, and the chronic fatigue syndrome is the most individual of diseases. Causes differ, symptoms vary, immune dysfunction fluctuates, and sensitivities, allergies and intolerance are as personally unique as are fingerprints. Obviously all these factors make treatment individual, too. What works for one may not work for another. The process of returning to health may take many months, even years. It will be a process of exploration and experimentation, disappointments and delight.

Since the immune system is too complex for simplistic remedies or 'magic bullets', more than one approach may be needed. Thus the choice of primary physician is crucial. Will he or she be able to see each patient as unique or individual? Does he or she believe in the reality of the chronic fatigue and immune dysfunction syndrome? Have some knowledge of nutrition and allergies? An understanding of alternative therapies? Will he or she be able to encourage patients to be independent, to have a sense of being in charge of their own destinies, and help them adopt a truly holistic approach to their health?

The relationship of CFS patients with the average busy GP is clouded from the start by the complexity of the symptoms. Any doctor who works on a 15-minute time frame simply cannot begin to understand a condition which may take two hours to explain. For a better chance of a helpful discussion, patients should try for consultations when the practice is not busy. Many CFS sufferers have come to know a considerable amount about their condition. They should remember, however, the old saying: 'There are two things a doctor doesn't like being told. One is something he doesn't know. The other is something he does.'

It is useful to make a list beforehand of main symptoms and questions for which answers are wanted, and then to note the answers. Memory impairment is a common CFS symptom – even the average patient remembers only about 20 per cent of information given during a consultation.

The importance of a holistic approach cannot be overstressed as the healing process may benefit from alternative approaches, particularly acupuncture, homoeopathy and exploration of the interaction between mind and body. Yet while every approach offers hope, and hopefully help, it is the combination of the strength of the relationship of the postively-minded patient and the open-minded physician that is most likely to achieve success.

How to start on this quest? This first step is to ask for a complete medical check-up that will focus on all possible causes for symptoms. If no cause is found, if the doctor's report is 'sound as a bell', and yet there is no improvement in vitality or symptoms, then this is the time to look for that exceptional primary physician who will give specialist treatment.

If the patient is philosophically inclined towards 'alternative' therapies, that move should be made at this point. Rather than providing a palliative treatment for symptoms, alternative therapies seek to provide a restorative approach to bring the patient to a higher level of health. Homoeopaths and acupuncturists, for instance, find it difficult both to diagnose and judge the effectiveness of their treatment when the natural expression of the patient's body has been distorted by palliative medications.

THE DOCTOR/PATIENT PARTNERSHIP

Any doctor intent on helping people overcome their M.E., chronic fatigue syndrome, candidiasis or allergies will soon have many patients. GPs specialising in this area usually have to close their books from time to time to catch up with the backlog of work. They are seeing people who have already made fruitless rounds of other doctors; patients from hundreds of miles away; patients who have been through every test possible for diseases ranging from brain tumours to arteriosclerosis, yet who are given an apparent clean bill of health every time.

The therapeutic approach of this admittedly small group of GPs has a holistic ring. It is firstly to unload the immune system of the most immediate burdens and secondly, to build up the patient's system by whatever approaches seem most appropriate.

The first step is to ascertain whether food intolerance and chemical sensitivities are causing immune dysfunction and digestive problems – in other words, assessing the patient's ecologic status. This is usually carried out with elimination dieting to ascertain food sensitivities, followed by rotational dieting to keep the burden low. Provocative neutralisation, in which tiny amounts of individual suspect substance are injected under the skin to form weals and cause physical reactions, is also used, particularly for foods causing Type 1 reactions (see Chapter 6, Allergies).

The doctor may also assess the patient's breathing, since hyper-ventilation – rapid, shallow, and often uncontrolled breathing – is associated with allergies in ways that are not really understood (possibly by upsetting the acid/alkali balance). Correct breathing often helps reduce allergic reactions.

About this time, perhaps two or three months from that first appointment, the possibility of starting a course of Enzyme Potenti-ated Desensitisation treatments may be discussed. As this is an option which is likely to cost the patient in excess of £500 over a two-year period, and appreciably more in Britain and the United States, it may not always be possible.

Because basic nutritional deficiencies are widespread in M.E. and CFS patients, the doctor may order nutritional assessments through hair, blood and sweat analyses. These will assess levels of B group vitamins which are all vital co-factors in metabolic pathways, of A,C,D,E which are important for immune health, of the essential fatty acids and amino acids and mineral trace element co-factors which are also essential to these processes.

If needed, nutritional supplementations will be advised. Since

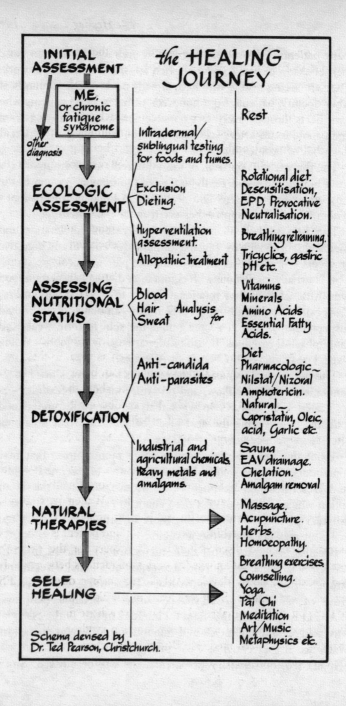

INITIAL ASSESSMENT

the HEALING JOURNEY

M.E. or chronic fatigue syndrome

other diagnosis

Rest

Intradermal/sublingual testing for foods and fumes.

ECOLOGIC ASSESSMENT

Exclusion Dieting.

Rotational diet. Desensitisation, EPD, Provocative Neutralisation.

Hyperventilation assessment.

Breathing retraining.

Allopathic treatment

Tricyclics, gastric pH etc.

ASSESSING NUTRITIONAL STATUS

Blood
Hair   Analysis
Sweat   for

Vitamins
Minerals
Amino Acids
Essential Fatty Acids.

Anti-candida
Anti-parasites

Diet
Pharmacologic –
Nilstat/Nizoral
Amphotericin.
Natural –
Capristatin, Oleic, acid, Garlic etc.

DETOXIFICATION

Industrial and agricultural chemicals. Heavy metals and amalgams.

Sauna
EAV drainage.
Chelation.
Amalgam removal

NATURAL THERAPIES

Massage.
Acupuncture.
Herbs.
Homoeopathy.

SELF HEALING

Breathing exercises.
Counselling.
Yoga.
Tai Chi
Meditation
Art/Music
Metaphysics etc.

Schema devised by Dr. Ted Pearson, Christchurch.

few of these receive prescription subsidies, they may be a great financial burden to the patient. Some patients are so sensitive that they can tolerate only special non-allergenic brands which may have to be imported.

By this time, most patients are feeling much, much better. Yet there will be some whose progress is disappointing in spite of the burdens unloaded, and the immune support being given. Possibly the immune system is being dragged down by residues of industrial chemicals, pesticides, fungal infections, parasites, heavy metals and dental amalgams. Blood samples may be sent overseas for analysis or a series of EAV tests may be carried out. A range of therapies may be recommended, from anti-candida diets and drugs, to homoeopathic drainage remedies, saunas, chelation therapy and amalgam removal and replacement.

It is usually at this stage that those who are vastly improved – maybe 70-85 per cent back to normal health – are encouraged to spread their wings and seek to tonify and balance their bodies through natural therapies such as massage, acupuncture, hydrotherapy, herbs and homoeopathy. From these therapies it is a short step to the healing arts of the East such as yoga, T'ai chi and meditation. Gentle exercise and swimming can be extremely helpful. Some patients learn to understand more about themselves and their illness through counselling, therapeutic art classes in the Steiner tradition, metaphysics and religion.

There will still be some sufferers who have faithfully followed these regimes and who still remain intractably ill. It is quite possible that tricyclic antidepressants, or therapies dealing with fundamental imbalances, such as those developed by doctors Emanuel Revici and Robert Erdmann and naturopaths like Walter Last, would provide sufficient correction for the healing process to continue.

The healing partnership between doctor and patient is a journey of exploration and discovery in which respect for the patient's individuality, and joint knowledge of the interactions between body and mind, are slowly developed. Like all chronic diseases, CFS teaches many lessons. Sufferers learn much along the way.

The options below make it clear that there is hope for people with the chronic fatigue and immune dysfunction syndrome. CFS is a challenge to Western medicine, and many doctors are working in the dark alongside their patients. More than with any other type of illness, CFS makes it necessary for the patient and the doctor to share education and beliefs.

Describing those patients who actively participate in their own recovery as 'exceptional', Bernie Siegel MD writes in *Love, Medicine and Miracles*: 'Exceptional patients refuse to be victims. They educate themselves and become specialists in their own care. They question the doctor because they want to understand their treatment and participate in it. They demand dignity, personhood, and control, no matter what the course of the disease.'

Those intent on returning to health should bear in mind:

• The need to work in partnership with the primary physician.
• Rest: CFS means that the whole system has been overloaded. Complete physical and mental rest if possible, and preferably from when symptoms first strike, will hasten recovery. When symptoms permit, regular gentle exercise (well within the boundaries of tolerance) such as walking, swimming, stretching exercises or simple yoga, is beneficial.
• An individualised version of the Pritikin or Stone Age diet (see Chapter 13). Recommended for all those with CFS are fresh organic foods and the avoidance of sugar, refined carbohydrates and fatty foods. Arginine-rich foods, which include peanuts, almonds and chocolate, are often not tolerated and should be avoided by those with herpesviruses.
• The avoidance of smoking and recreational drugs; alcohol only occasionally, then in very small quantities (none if candida is a problem).
• The avoidance, wherever possible, of all steroid drugs (Prednisone especially), and sprays such as Aldecin, Becotide and Beconase; all oral contraceptives, antibiotics, particularly the broad spectrum drugs and tetracyclines, and, for the salicylate-sensitive, avoidance of drugs containing salicylates, such as aspirin.
• Medicinal herbs and homoeopathic remedies – these should be used only with the guidance of a properly trained herbalist, naturopath or acupuncturist.

HEALING APPROACHES (listed alphabetically)

Note that these are intended to show that there are many options open to both doctor and patient, but in no way are they a grab-bag for casual sampling without professional guidance. They are not of equal importance, and many will not be available in a particular district or country. None is guaranteed; each may help some, and be useless to others. They represent the state of the art in mid-1988, to the best knowledge of many specialists.

Finding what is most helpful to the individual is often a matter of trial and error. As each individual's illness develops and changes in its nature, what works at one stage may be useless at another. Patients should not ring the changes on their treatment without guidance and should remain in close consultation with their doctor. The letters (Pr) following a drug name mean that it is obtainable on prescription only; the letters (DA) mean that the treatment or substance in question is usually administered by a doctor though some may be administered by a chiropractor, acupuncturist, homoeopath or naturopath (who may also be a doctor). Preparations without letters following are available from chemists, health food shops, or specialist suppliers.

ALLERGIES – DIAGNOSIS (AND TREATMENTS)
Five-day fasts, followed by the gradual introduction of foods, were the principal method of determining food allergies. This approach, however, often left patients with more allergies than before. Elimination dieting is less stressful. See next chapter. The following methods are quicker, have fewer side effects, but may not be as reliable.

The Provocative-Neutralisation test (DA) Small amounts of different dilutions of the antigen are squirted under the tongue or injected under the skin to produce symptoms (such as chills, tachycardia, dizziness, etc). The correct dilution is reached when the reactions no longer occur. The patient is then supplied with drops at the dilution to take as required. The drops (antigen therapy) can turn off allergic reactions as well as preventing them. They gradually build up immunity, and many people have no need for them after about a year. This is a standard and widely available approach which is excellent for inhalant allergens. Best results occur when the patient has only a few major allergies.

Electroacupuncture (DA) Using bio-electrical equipment, the physician diagnoses allergies by measuring electrical reactions in the patient's body to phials containing homoeopathic potencies of allergens. The method (electroacupuncture according to Voll) is more fully described on p.100. It is extremely rapid, has no side effects whatsoever, but is not always reliable. The skill, intuition and medical knowledge of the operator is crucial. Following diagnosis, appropriate steps (such as avoidance and rotational dieting) can be taken. Operators claim about 80 per cent success in diagnosis and treatments. See Bio-energetic Regulatory Medicine, p.100.

Applied Kinesiology (DA) Used by chiropractors and holistic therapists. The patient's muscle strength is tested with different foods and chemicals. Muscle strength is weaker on exposure to allergens. When the allergens are discovered, therapy can proceed.

Pulse testing The pulse is taken before eating or before sublingual drops of mashed food or food extract.Then it is taken five, ten and thirty minutes afterwards. A marked acceleration or deceleration signals an allergic reaction. Symptoms may be switched off by taking Tri-salts or a teaspoon of bicarbonate of soda in a glass of warm water.

Cytotoxic testing A laboratory test to determine allergies. It involves assessing the inhibition of movement and break-up of white cells before and after the addition of weak solutions of antigens. It is reasonably reliable when carried out by an experienced technician in a reputable laboratory, but is expensive and not always available.

Urine tests with ultraviolet light A blue tinge will show up when urine containing proteins caused by food intolerances is exposed to UV light. (A reddish-purple tinge is shown in the urine of porphyrics.) A quick and simple test with many applications.

ALLERGIES – treatment only
Enzyme Potentiated Desensitisation (DA) A medical procedure developed in 1966 by Dr Len McEwen at St Mary's Hospital, Paddington, London. He found that an enzyme, beta glucuronidase, could be used to potentiate the effect of an injection of grass

pollen extract for hay fever. A single shot was as effective as a long course of traditional injections.

Dr McEwen has adapted EPD to treat other allergies. Minute quantities of food allergens, pollens, house dusts and animal dander (more than 60 substances, some cross-reacting) are injected sub-cutaneously. Treatments have a cumulative effect, and though initially given every two months, are then given at longer intervals. They are expensive because of production costs of the vaccine, and the need for nutritional supplementation.

During the period 1983–6 Dr Belinda Dawes of London developed a regime to maximise the effect of EPD. This includes testing for food allergies and vitamin and mineral deficiencies; anti-candida therapy; and the prescription of relevant nutritional supplementation. These measures, in association with EPD, enable CFS sufferers to recover more quickly. More than 80 per cent of patients show marked improvements in health.

In spite of the success rate, Dr McEwen stresses that the best treatment for food allergy is simple avoidance. Only when sensitivity is so extreme to a substance which is so widespread it is difficult to avoid, or when an individual has so many food intolerances that a balanced diet is impossible, should EPD be considered.

(Dr McEwen says EPD is a useful treatment for bedwetting when all other approaches have failed. One treatment appears to provide a permanent cure.)

EPD treatments are available in the United Kingdom, the United States, Italy, Germany and New Zealand. Their originator, Dr McEwen, holds periodic training seminars for doctors, and has produced a technical booklet. (Dr L.H. McEwen, Weir View, Wargrave Road, Henley-on-Thames, Oxon, England.)

Chiropractic (DA) The theory of chiropractic is that misaligned vertebrae obstruct the flow of nerve energy, and when the vertebrae are realigned, symptoms including allergic reactions, inexplicable pain, fatigue, headaches and muscle spasms are reduced. There is a strong connection between the central nervous system and allergies, and CFS has a major neurological component.

Amino acids Glycine, cysteine, glutamic acid and histadine taken with selenium, vitamins B6 and C. Also see under Nutritional Supplementation.

Sodium chloride irrigation solution. Squirted into nostrils night and morning, this will loosen mucus and clear out allergens in the nasal passages. No side effects. The mucus flows into the mouth and is then expectorated.

Tri-salts A useful 'sipping solution' to turn off bad Type 2 reactions. 3 parts sodium bicarbonate; 2 parts potassium bicarbonate; 1 part calcium carbonate. Mix 1 level tsp with 1 large cup of cold water. Stir frequently and sip slowly during the day. If too strong, or taken too quickly, may cause looseness of bowels. Has also been found to energise weak, aching muscles.

Digestive enzymes Pancreatic and gastric enzyme preparations aid digestion so that undigested and partially digested protein fractions are less likely to pass through the walls of the digestive tract. This may reduce reaction severity.

Sodium Cromoglycate (Pr) This stabilises mast cells in the gut and reduces allergic reactions. Trade names are Nalcrom for food allergy, and Intal, principally for asthma. Nalcrom is taken 4 times a day before meals, 100mg for children; 200mg for adults. This is useful to allow an occasional dietary lapse as at Christmas and birthdays, but is not recommended on a long-term basis. Intal, 5 capsules a day.

Autoimmune urine therapy Sub-lingual drops of a 1-in-5 dilution of the patient's urine, collected at a reaction peak, administered under the tongue; 3-6 drops four times a day. This has been found very useful by some; useless by others. Possibly the difficulties of remembering to collect at a true reaction peak may affect results.

Transfer factor A material extracted from the white blood cells of healthy donors. A series of injections may remove or reduce allergies. Dr Alan Levin (U.S.A.) reports a 76 per cent success rate.

Anti-histamines Use with great caution. Terfenedine (Teldane) (Pr) and Hismanal (Pr) have been found helpful for the typical Type 1 reactions such as stuffy noses and streaming eyes. Homoeopathically prepared histamines are used for their anti-histamine effect and appear safe enough in low potencies.

Also possibly helpful: magnetic therapy as advised by Dr W.M. Philpott, and removal of mercury amalgam fillings by a specialist dental practitioner.

BOOKS TO READ:

Allergies ... what everyone should know, by Keith Mumby, Unwin Paperbacks, 1986.
Chemical Victims, by Dr Richard Mackarness, Pan Books, 1980.
Allergies, Your Hidden Enemy, by Theron Randolph and Dr Ralph Moss, Turnstone Press, U.K., 1980.
Dr Mandell's 5 Day Allergy Relief System, by Dr Marshall Mandell, Arrow Books, 1983.
New Hope for Physical and Emotional Illnesses: Values of magnetic energy and oxygen, by W.H. Philpott, Enviro-Tech Products, U.S.A., 1987.

ANXIETY

Stress reduction therapies, meditation and increased exercise (where possible) should be the first steps taken to reduce anxiety or heart palpitations. Then, if these fail or are not acceptable to the patient:

The monoamine oxidase inhibitors (MAO inhibitors) (Pr). Particularly Parnate (Pr) and Nardil (Pr) can be helpful, but need to be used with great care. They improve the brain's biochemical functioning and restore cell and mitochondrial respiratory function in muscles and nervous system. With possible dangerous side-effects, they should be taken only in conjunction with a strictly amine-free diet. The benzodiazepines are not recommended for these symptoms.

Anti-stress nutritional supplementation. May be helpful in conjunction with other approaches.

Amino acid therapy. As the use of amino acid supplementation is becoming more widespread, there are numerous reports from both doctors and patients of its success in improving brain functioning and reducing depression and anxiety. Dr Robert Erdmann recommends an amino formula of tryptophan (NOT in conjunction with MAO inhibitors), histidine, glycine, taurine and co-factors vitamins B1, B2, B6, calcium ascorbate, vitamin C and zinc.

Magnetic therapy has been found helpful by some. See under special heading.

BACTERIA AND PARASITES
See under Digestive Problems and Candida.

BODY BALANCING
The forces that maintain the body's homoeostatic balance may be compared with the positive/negative opposing but complementary forces that run through the universe.

When the metabolism (the production of energy within the cells) is disrupted, the cells may become either over-acid or over-alkaline. Increased muscle cell lactic acid is, for example, a feature in CFS, with accompanying decreases in nerve energy and muscle strength. Symptoms of systemic overalkalinity include wounds that are slow to heal, and being consistently several pounds lighter in the morning than at night.

Over-acidity of the system (blood, tissues and urine) and under-acidity of the stomach is a basis for poor digestion and fatigue, and may lead on to more serious conditions.

Correction of these imbalances, of acid/alkaline, sodium/potassium, and catabolic/anabolic, has provided relief for allergies and many other chronic conditions. Rapid cures and relief of muscle weakness have been brought about by such simple (yet innately sophisticated) approaches as drinking large amounts of slightly salty water. Doctors and nutritionists following Dr Revici's methods (see Chapter 5) also report some real successes, along with the disappointments.

Macrobiotic doctors recommend eating less and chewing well; hot foot baths; alternate hot and cold showers; Do-In massage (slapping the body briskly); plenty of salads and alkaline-forming foods; yoga breathing; walking and gardening.

Other useful therapeutic approaches are magnetic therapy, amino acids, acupuncture and naturopathy. Also see Digestive Problems.

This is an area for research, experimentation and discovery.

RECOMMENDED READING
Acid and Alkaline, by Herman Aihara, Nutri-Books Corp, U.S.A., 1980.
Brain Allergies: the psycho-nutrient connection, by Wm H. Philpott and Dwight K. Kalita, Keats Publishing Inc, U.S.A., 1980.
Heal Yourself, by Walter Last, Nelson Aust., 1984.

CANDIDA – anti-candida agents with few side effects
The importance of following an anti-candida diet during treatment cannot be over-emphasised. Ridding the body of fungal overgrowth is a challenging procedure. Some people are able to knock it out quickly, while for others it may take many months of experimenting with different forms of treatment before improvement is seen.

Nystatin (Pr) (also called Mycostatin, Nilstat) One of the safest drugs available, it is the most common treatment for candida, and receives most favourable comment of all anti-fungal agents. It has been reported that, along with reducing the symptoms of CFS, it has helped many other conditions. Among them are: depression, manic-depression, psoriasis, dermatitis, asthma, multiple sclerosis (effective in restoring bladder control), allergies, rheumatoid arthritis, irritable bowel syndrome, hyperactivity and 'glue-ear'. Even persistent bad breath has been helped by Nystatin treatment.

Start with 1 tablet four times daily; after two weeks, 2 tablets four times daily; after another two weeks, up to 18 tablets a day in divided doses. May need to be taken for several years. For skin conditions, use the cream; for oral thrush, the liquid; for vaginal thrush, use pessaries or tampons soaked in a Nystatin solution.

The powder is preferable where the mouth, throat and upper digestive area are affected. For the duodenum, Nilstat tablets; for colon overgrowth, use Mycostatin tablets. Nystatin powder enemas are also helpful.

ANZMES (N.Z.) suggests that, for a full trial of the benefits of Nystatin, the patient should work up to 16 tablets or two teaspoonsful of powder a day. If the problem is suspected to be throughout the gastro-intestinal tract, from mouth to rectum, the following is recommended: 1 tsp pure powder daily, 8 Nilstat tablets daily, 8 tablets Mycostatin daily.

If the problem is in the mouth, the powder should be taken after meals and preferably after brushing the teeth and tongue. Some powder should be mixed in the mouth with saliva and spread around the mouth. Disregard the taste.

The major drawback with Nystatin is its effectiveness. It kills yeast cells in such numbers that they release sufficient toxic substances to produce a temporary toxic-like condition. This is called the Herxheimer reaction or burnoff. This can be reduced by having a low-carbohydrate diet beforehand.

There is a small percentage of patients who have a genuine allergic reaction to the Nystatin itself.

Immunotherapy (DA) Anti-candida vaccines and antigenic extracts are effective for some, but can produce brain reactions. Skin tests can be given to assess reactivity. Not usually suitable for people with autoimmune manifestations or who are already taking Nystatin. The homoeopathic dilution is usually 30C.

Canestan – clotrimazole (Pr) Tablets, vaginal cream, solution or pessaries.

Nizoral – ketoconazole (Pr) An effective systemic anti-fungal agent used for sytemic and deep infections. With possible serious side effects (principally liver damage), it should be closely monitored, and it should be used only as a last resort.

Amphotericin B, Fungilin or Fungizone (Pr) In creams, lotions and ointments for skin and mucous membrane candida. Taken orally in tablets or powdered form penetrates deeply into the gut wall (may cause diarrhoea).

An alternative approach Growing attention is being paid to approaches which do not use anti-yeast medications. They consist of:

(a) Reinoculating the bowel with bacterial supplements These products are seeded with the human intestinal lactobacilli and are a natural way to control candida in the gut. They also suppress staphylococci and prevent or alleviate antibiotic-induced diarrhoea. Various types of lactobacillus acidophilus include Orthodophilus (lactose-free); Vitaldophilus (for milk-sensitive people); Superdophilus, particularly powerful, and new versions, such as Vitalplex, containing other bacteria. Special unsweetened yoghurts are available seeded with lactobacilli, and can either be eaten or used as a vaginal douche.

(b) Supplementation to prevent the candida from converting from the yeast form to the invasive form 300 mcg biotin taken three times daily and two tsp olive oil taken three times daily. The latter is a source of oleic acid. Diet should have a higher than normal fibre content, particularly oat bran.

Caprylic acid Capricin, Caprystatin, Capricidin and Candistat-300 are related preparations available for oral and vaginal use. A fatty acid derived from coconut oil, it works by smothering the fungus. Should not be used by people allergic to coconut.

(c) Supplementation to heal the mucosa of the intestinal tract once the organism has been arrested in its growth Zinc, 30-50mg daily; vit E, 400-800 IUs daily; calcium pantothenate, 200-1000mg daily.

Other Approaches:

Enemas Nystatin enemas (following a standard enema) are recommended for lower bowel overgrowth. They have about a teaspoon of Nystatin powder to a quart of warm purified water and may also be used for a vaginal douche and can be used daily.

Vaginal douches Pure unsweetened yoghurt, either full strength or diluted with pure water; tampons soaked in vinegar, medicated aloe vera gel, or liquid garlic and left in overnight; lactobacillus acidophilus powder (½ tsp to 1½ cups water); sorbic acid: Orithrush-D and Orifresh; capsule evening primrose oil.

Hydrogen peroxide 35% food grade, 1-3 drops in 5oz water, 3 times a day is the starting dose. Increase by a drop per dose per day. Drink first thing in the morning at least 30 minutes before food. Also last thing at night. A hydrogen peroxide gargle helps oral thrush. Dilution should be 1 part to 5 or 10 parts water (do not drink). Dilute further if too strong. Boosts energy, controls parasites and bacteria. Though the possibility of free radical enhancement would seem a strong reason why H_2O_2 should not be used, this recommendation comes from California therapists working with AIDS and other immune dysfunction illnesses.

Gentian violet Used for painting fungal lesions on skin, mouth and perineal areas.

Iodine therapy If candida symptoms are accompanied by lumpy breasts, nutritional physician Jonathon Wright, MD of Seattle recommends painting the vaginal area with iodine about once every six months. Magnesium sulphate should be injected following the iodine treatment. This stimulates the ovaries and improves endocrine balance. Iodine-rich nutritional supplementation of kelp, iodine tablets, etc should be given or paint the soles of the feet with iodine.

Herbal teas Lapacho, Pau d'Arco or taheebo tea is found useful by some; Mathake tea from Fiji, reputedly a very powerful anti-fungal agent; cherry bark; gingseng and goldenseal. Chapparal tea is especially recommended: from 1 tsp to 1 tbs chapparal to one quart of water; bring to the boil, and steep below boiling temperature for 30 to 60 minutes. Sweeten with boiled honey, if desired. Use all these in consultation with a herbalist.

Garlic (fresh Kyolic or Pure-Gar) Extremely effective against candida and persistant bacteria. Considered by many to be the most effective anti-fungal agent of all. Deodorised commercial preparations do not have the penetrating garlic odour.

Australian tea tree oil (only from *Melaleuca alternifolia*) Highly recommended by California AIDS therapists. Work up to 6 drops 3 times daily.

Herbs A naturopath will recommend effective ways of using thyme, cinnamon, cloves, eucalyptus, and mustard, all of which are recognised for their anti-fungal properties. Oriental medicine also offers a range of anti-fungal herbs.

Sorbic acid This fatty acid derived from the berries of the American mountain ash is particularly effective against fungal infections. Orithrush-G (for gargling) and Orithrush-D (for douching) are the preparations most widely available.

BOOKS TO READ:

The Yeast Connection (revised edition), by Dr William Crook,

Professional Books, 1987.
The Yeast Syndrome, by Leslie Trowbridge and Dr Morton Walker, Bantam, 1986.

COUNSELLING

Talking over problems with a counsellor who is experienced in dealing with people with chronic illness may be one of the most helpful things a patient can do. Many need to come to terms with changes in relationships, finances, careers. There is often also a need to come to terms with grief and anger sometimes arising from childhood traumas, and work out ways to change attitudes that are unhelpful to the healing process. A counsellor who is alert to the body/mind connection may also be able to help individuals strengthen their immune systems through the power of their minds.

CYSTITIS

Urine should first be checked by a laboratory for the presence of infectious agents. If present, then antibiotic treatment is usual. Cystitis can be caused by allergies (usually in conjunction with candida) which inflame the bladder and urethra. If no infections are found, the possibility of hidden allergies should be explored, and steps taken to avoid those foods causing trouble, and to treat candida. Extreme sexual and perineal hygiene should be practised.

At the onset of an attack, a glass of water or a bland drink (such as 1 tbs barley cooked till it bursts, cooled, strained, flavoured with lemon juice, diluted with water) should be drunk every twenty minutes for three hours. Sipping Tri-Salts or taking Cymalon every three hours helps correct acidity.

Cystitis sufferers have discovered a virtue of couch grass (twitch). A tea made from its well-simmered runners is extremely soothing.

BOOKS TO READ

Understanding Cystitis – a complete self-help guide, by Angela Kilmartin, Century Arow, 1985.
Victims of Thrush and Cystitis, by Angela Kilmartin, Century Arrow, 1986.

DEPRESSION – anti-depressants for CFS patients

Many people with CFS reject the idea of taking anti-depressants, considering this implies their illness is only of the mind. Yet anti-depressants affect the whole body in a number of ways. The tricyclic group of anti-depressants may be specially helpful (see Chapter 11). The way they work is not clearly understood, but it is thought to relate to anti-inflammatory properties, to enzyme induction of important neurotransmitters in the brain, and effects on smooth muscle.

Tricyclics seem to cause fewer side effects, significantly reduce pain, improve sleep, and are less addictive than other types of anti-depressants. Dosage may need to be increased very slowly and maintained for several weeks before full benefits are seen.

Amino acid therapy Dr Erdmann recommends L-phenylalanine, tyrosine, and methionine taken 3 times daily with magnesium, vitamins B1, B3, B6, C and zinc. Tyrosine and L-phenylalanine should not be taken in conjunction with MAO inhibitors. These essential nutrients are also involved in the synthesis of neurotransmitters and should not be overlooked.

Monoamine oxidase inhibitors (Pr) Start at 15 mg daily for a week, then increase dosage to 30-45-60mg daily. For fuller details, see under Anxiety.

When all else has failed, some fine help from benzodiazepine (Pr) (especially Doxiepam or Ativan). There is a possibility of addiction.

Magnetic Therapy as outlined by Dr Philpott may also be helpful (see under Magnetic Therapy).

DETOXIFICATION

Toxins can take many forms in the body; viral, fungal, bacterial, chemical and metals. Removal will be more difficult if the toxins have moved from the extra-cellular fluids to within the cells (particularly chemicals in fat cells). Persistent toxins usually indicate cellular breakdown and liver damage. Every effort should be made to improve overall cellular health through superior nutrition, and by supporting and regenerating the liver and kidneys. Once their function is improved, toxins may disappear naturally from the body.

For serious toxic burdens, there are a number of approaches:

Natural detoxifying agents Vitamin C in massive amounts: helps revitalise damaged cell walls; increases the effectiveness of liver enzymes that detoxify pesticides and other chemicals; attaches to mineral molecules and is then excreted. Some people find help from Swedish Bitters, a herbal mixture. Linseed and olive oils will pick up fat-soluble toxins. Used as laxatives, they help remove chemicals by bonding with them and removing them from the body. Aloe vera juice has similar properties. Activated charcoal: an old remedy, this one – often effective and often overlooked. Hydrogen peroxide in very weak dilutions; hyperbaric oxygen treatment is a helpful adjunct.

Homoeopathic approaches Drainage remedies (homoepathic dilutions of toxins) are useful to expel toxins from within the cells to the extra-cellular fluid. These are then excreted from the body through the digestive and urinary systems and the skin.

Saunas plus natural detoxifying agents Those specialising in the treatment of CFS will do themselves and their patients a favour by installing a sauna and providing supervised detoxification regimes. Dr Doug Seba and other U.S. specialists speak highly of the success of this approach in removing viral and chemical toxins.

Variations on the following regime are being used successfully by a number of detoxification centres such as Human Environmental Medicine of San Diego (see p. 81); 15-30 minutes' brisk exercise, up to 4 hours daily in a dry sauna with hourly breaks for fluids, plus large amounts of vitamins in incremental doses. These include A, B-complex, niacin, niacinamide, C, D and E, plus amino acids (particularly cysteine), linseed oil or olive oil, and multiminerals including calcium and magnesium.

Though saunas should be as hot as possible, their heat and length should be adjusted to the vitality of the individual. There is a difference of opinion as to which is most effective – dry or moist saunas. Weight should be maintained during this type of detoxification. Fat consumption should be lowered, and special care taken to avoid any foods containing pesticides, synthetic hormones or antibiotics.

Metal chelators – oral There is a number of newly developed oral chelators now appearing on the market. They apparently have fewer side effects than EDTA. Most are in tablet form. One that may be useful is DMPS (Di-mercapto-propane-sulphonate), a German product which is said to cross the blood/brain barrier.

EDTA chelation This is an intravenous chelation process by which metals or minerals in the body are bonded to a man-made amino acid called Ethylene-diamine-tetra-acetate.

A.N.Z.M.E.S. reports that as presently used, it is not helpful for CFS patients, and unpleasant side-effects have been reported. Nevertheless, it may have a place as a same-day back-up to mercury amalgam removal.

BOOKS TO READ:

Detox, by Phyllis Saifer and Merla Zellerbach, Ballantine Books, N.Y., 1984.
The Miracle Healing Power of Chelation Therapy, by Dr Morton Walker, Fischer Pubs, U.S., 1984.

DIGESTIVE PROBLEMS

The overgrowth of candida and other intestinal bacteria, plus the ingestion of foods to which the individual is intolerant (particularly cow's milk) are major factors in creating ongoing digestive problems through damage to the walls of the gut. Liver and pancreatic damage is also a contributing factor to digestive problems. Lower than normal levels of hydrochloric acid in the stomach are now thought to set in train a long list of gastrointestinal disorders, including candida overgrowth, which lead on to other problems.

The term dysbiosis is used in BER medicine to describe overall digestive dysfunction caused by abnormal intestinal bacteria. Symptoms include flatulence, disordered bowel habit, and intermittent abdominal swelling. Dysbiosis may lead to irritable bowel syndrome, spastic colon, ulcerative colitis, and even Crohn's disease.

Fungal infections, bacteria and parasites in the digestive system need to be treated in ways that enhance, rather than depress the immune system. Though they may be effective, most prescription drugs have serious side effects. The safest approaches are the natural ones which encourage the body to repair itself. These include correcting the stomach and gut pH, using digestive enzymes to improve the quality of digestion, and boosting with amino acids to help gut membranes and other organs repair themselves.

Treatment of allergies with appropriate diet regimes is vital to improved digestion. Though elimination dieting is not recommended because of the already poor nutritional status of patients, it is often very helpful to avoid cow's milk and all dairy products, meats (particularly red meats), sugar and refined carbohydrates, gluten, grain and eggs. The best diet is low-fat vegetarian. Since nutrient absorption is reduced, a broad range of supplementation, including digestive enzymes, should be considered. Magnesium deficiencies are particularly likely following chronic diarrhoea, which often benefits from an amino acid anxiety formula.

A high fibre diet incorporating plenty of fresh fruit and vegetables and fruits is an important aspect of regularising bowel movements. Preparations such as Isogel can also be helpful. Bowel cleaning can be achieved with psyllium husks, prune and senna tablets, and a Gastrobrom/Pascopancreat (U.S.) mixture for general digestion.

Amino acid therapy Dr Robert Erdmann recommends glutamic acid HCL, trytophan (not in conjunction with MAO inhibitors), histidine, glycine, betaine HCL and co-factors vitamins B3, B6, and ascorbic acid.

Anti-parasitical herbal mixture: A San Francisco holistic group, working with people with AIDS, recommends the following: 1 cup dried cabbage leaves, ½ cup Kyolic garlic, ⅓ cup Korean gingseng, ⅓ cup organically grown tobacco. Take 2 tbs twice daily separated by at least six hours. Even more effective when 1-2 large cups of sauerkraut is eaten daily.

Homoeopathy 'drainage' treatments These help the body excrete toxins from bacteria and parasites.

Sulphonamides Are effective in toxoplasmosis, with few side effects.

High doses of PABA, magnetic therapy and mercury amalgam removal have also been found to be helpful. 2-6 drops of peppermint oil per meal have also helped candida-related symptoms and general intestinal irritation.

BOOKS TO READ:
Detox, by Dr Phyllis Saifer and Merla Zellerbach, Ballantine Books, 1984.

HOMOEOPATHY

Classical homoeopathic medicine is a blend of extremely detailed diagnosis and pharmaceutics. It uses minute amounts of various plant, mineral, animal, bacterial, viral and chemical preparations to stimulate the sick person's natural defences. It is often effective for chronic immune dysfunction disease because it works by building up the body and its immune defences, rather than suppressing symptoms. The remedies chosen for each individual relate to the pattern of symptoms, to the organs most affected and to the personality of the patient. Skilled homoeopaths are on record as stimulating the healing process with a single dose of a single remedy, and people with CFS have been known to regain their full health along with a better emotional balance in as few as four months.

Homoeopaths find it difficult to diagnose patients who have already been treated with various medications and nutritional supplements. If homoeopathy is considered, it is therefore wise to consult a homoeopath early in the search for health, and after conventional medical testing has established no other causes for ill health.

HYPOGLYCAEMIA

Fluctuating and low blood sugar levels are an important cause of a Pandora's box of multiple confusing symptoms. Assessing whether hypoglycaemia is their cause is such a complex and time-consuming business that, in practice, testing for blood sugar levels tends to be reserved for diabetics only.

A 12-hour fast is required before taking the Glucose Tolerance Test and a blood sample is then taken to determine the fasting blood sugar level. Then a glucose drink is given followed by further blood samples at specific intervals. Testing should be on an extended basis, of at least 8 hours. If blood sugar levels fail to rise by at least 50mg per cent above the fasting blood sugar mark, or if they drop more than 20 mg below, and if symptoms occur which correlate with blood sugar drops, then a diagnosis of hypoglycaemia can be made.

See Chapter 13 (Nutritional Approaches) for an outline of dietary changes that are needed to stabilise blood sugar levels.

Supplementation Dr Stephen Davies recommends: Tryptophan supplementation, 500-150mg daily; niacinamide supplementation, 1000-3000mg daily (with liver function testing every couple of months); B complex vitamins, 20-100mg daily; chromium GFT 200mcg daily; zinc, 15-25mg daily; manganese, 5-10mg daily; magnesium, 200-400mg daily; potassium, 500-1000mg daily, vitamin C, 2000-3000mg daily.

BOOKS TO READ:
Nutritional Medicine, by Drs Stephen Davies and Alan Stewart, Pan Books, 1987.
Low Blood Sugar and You, by Carlton Fredericks and Herman Goodman, Charter paperback, Grosset & Dunlop, 1969.
A Natural Approach to Diabetes and Hypoglycaemia, by Michio Kushi, Japan Pubs Inc, 1985.

IMMUNE-ENHANCING AND SYMPTOM-REDUCING AGENTS
Mostly expensive; often helpful, but no guarantee of effectiveness.
Vitamin C Orally or can be administered intravenously.
Amino acids A generalised amino acid supplementation provides the basic nutrients on which the immune system is constructed.
Coenzyme Q-10 or Ubiquinone A coenzyme in oxygen transfer, it increases levels of IgG, stimulates thymus, improves energy levels in impaired cells, helps heart muscles repair. Not where hypersensitivity is pronounced. If there is no improvement after three weeks, discontinue. May be available only in the United States.
Organic germanium – germanium sesquioxide: This stimulates the immune system, oxygenates the cells, is beneficial against candida and other pathogens. Is thought to act as a semi-conductor because of the way it strengthens the body's energetic forces.
Glandular extracts Thymus, pituitary, adrenals, thyroid, ovaries, etc – may boost underactive endocrine glands. Use only under direction.
Homoeopathic thymus preparation A useful preparation which normalises thymus function. Again, to be taken only under direction.
Acupuncture (DA) Strengthens and balances the body's energies and organs.
Oxygen-saturated Aloe Vera Californian clinician Dr Kurt

Donsbach manufactures this, and describes it as detoxifying, immune-boosting and healing.

Blue-Green Manna A single-cell algae, rich in chlorophyll and the eight essential amino-acids, vitamins, minerals and lipids. Appears to rejuvenate the thymus gland, the spleen and other factors of the immune system. Claimed to energise the brain, and contribute to cellular stability in the body. Recommended highly by holistic practitioners dealing with AIDS. Also the very similar Sun Chlorella, a Japanese product.

Attention to dental fillings Dental fillings, particularly those containing mercury, may be a factor in depressing the immune system. They should be evaluated with a view to replacement by a less reactive substance only by a dentist skilled in this area.

Intramuscular gamma globulin (DA) Concentration of anti-bodies found in blood, has high proportion of IgG, replaces deficient antibodies. An immune modulator, also helpful for viral and bacterial infections, especially for those with IgG deficiency (hypogammaglobulinaemia). Good rate of success with intravenous use. It had bad initial publicity in the United Kingdom because of AIDS contamination, but this is no longer a problem.

Isoprinosine (DA) A synthetic immune strengthening agent which increases NK cell activity, helper T cell count and helper/suppressor ratio. Still in the proving stages.

Thymosin (DA) A thymus extract which specifically affects the T cells and rejuvenates the spleen. A most effective American AIDS treatment, supplies still limited. Administered intravenously.

Transfer factor (DA) A material extracted from the white blood cells of healthy donors, it strengthens T cells and enhances immunity. Very expensive; needs to be taken fortnightly for about six months.

Also possibly useful are Shiitake mushroom extracts, Chinese tonifying herbs, pollen and echinacea.

BOOKS TO READ:

Include those recommended under Allergies and Viruses.

It's All In Your Head (Diseases Caused by Silver-Mercury Fillings), by Hal Huggins and S.A. Huggins, available from P.O. Box 2589, Colorado Springs, CO 80901, USA.

MAGNETIC THERAPY

Magnetic therapy is one of the 'suspect' healing approaches in that it is still little known. Dr W.H. Philpott, co-author of *Brain Allergies*, recommends magnetic therapy and breathing techniques for the treatment of allergies, addictions, nervous conditions, cuts, burns and bruises, infections, toxic conditions and general metabolic disorders. Medical magnets are approved by the Japanese Health Department and are widely used in Japanese hospitals for a variety of complaints. Magnetic therapy, in conjunction with correct breathing, appears to improve and balance the body's energies, and may be particularly helpful with catabolic/anabolic imbalances. It is important to see only a really skilled and knowledgeable therapist (addresses are given in Appendix 6).

Medical magnets have a south pole side and a north pole side. The north pole application is recommended for nearly all conditions, including CFS.

The magnetic polarity response differential is summarised as:

North Pole	South Pole
Produces alkanity in biological systems.	Produces acidity. Speeds up infection which can override
Slows down infections (viruses, bacteria, fungi) and aids metabolic defence against infections.	metabolic defences against infections.
Reduces pain.	Increases pain.
Reduces inflammation	Increases inflammation
Pulls fluid towards magnet	Repels fluid
Controlling effect on the brain	Disorganising effect.

RECOMMENDED READING:

The Magnetic Effect, by A.R.Davis and W. Rawls, Exposition Press, N.Y., 1975.
Basics of Food Allergy, by J. Breneman, 2nd ed. Charles C. Thomas, Springfield, Ill., 1984. pp 26, 168-9, 192, 222.
New Hope for Physical and Emotional Illnesses: Values of Magnetic

Energy and Oxygen, by W.H. Philpott, Enviro-Tech Products, 1987.

MENSTRUAL AND FEMALE
REPRODUCTIVE SYSTEM PROBLEMS
These include the pre-menstrual syndrome, pelvic inflammatory disease, endometriosis and painful periods.

While hormonal treatment is often helpful, the possibility of candida overgrowth should not be overlooked. If it is present, as it probably will be, symptoms may show a marked improvement after treatment both with diet and medications. Increased exercise and avoidance of smoking are also important.

Supplementations recommended are: Evening primrose oil, blackcurrant oil and codliver oil which all provide Omega-3 fatty acids. Linseed oil and lecithin provide Omega-6 fatty acids. All are helpful in correcting hormonal imbalances.

NUTRITIONAL SUPPLEMENTS
Individual needs for CFS patients vary enormously, and testing by hair, sweat or serum analysis should be carried out before recommendations are made. *Any supplementation should be taken under the supervision of a knowledgeable physician or naturopath.* Low levels of vitamin C, B12, zinc, iron, selenium and sometimes cobalt, chromium and manganese are often seen in patients. Supplements should preferably be free from yeast, wheat, gluten, milk, corn, soya, artificial colourings and preservatives. The normal dietary intake should be included in the following recommendations. (Supplements particularly useful for candida treatment are shown in italics.)

Testing for nutritional deficiencies To avoid guesses as to an individual's nutritional status, a proper analysis of vitamin, mineral, trace element and amino and fatty acid levels should be carried out.

Laboratories in the USA, UK and Australia test hair, blood or sweat samples. Tests are expensive, but they do enable recommendations to be tailored to individual needs, and may save money in the long term.

Supplements – amino acids A general amino acid mix, such as Pro-amino-plex, improves immunity and reduces stress and depression. Amino acids are now being recommended by nutritionally-oriented doctors.

Supplements – essential fatty acids *Evening primrose oil or linseed oil (both Omega 6 EFAs)* up to 2,000mg daily; *cod liver oil, an Omega 3 fatty acid (Twin Labs or Dale Alexander's brands); oleic acid (from olive oil).* Note that these must not be allowed to become rancid. Take one dessertspoonful of one oil only per day. *Aloe vera juice* (contains several EFAs) one dsp in water twice daily.

Supplements – mineral and trace elements Iron (chelated) (Pr), up to 60 mg (must not be taken with tea or coffee); *elemental zinc (Pr)*, up to 50mg daily preferably taken apart from other mineral supplementation; *selenium* (up to 50mcg daily, vital for enzyme functioning, useful in detoxification, enhances oxygenation and bio-energies); *iodine (kelp)*, 1-3 tablets daily; elemental calcium, (Pr), up to 2gms daily, elemental magnesium, (Pr), up to 50mg daily; elemental chromium, up to 100mg daily; manganese, up to 10mg daily; germanium (enhances oxygenation and bio-energies) up to 250mg daily; effervescent potassium chloride, 10mg daily. (Pr).

Supplements – vitamins *Vit A* up to 10,000 IUs daily; all B vitamins, (Pr), as directed, *vit B6* (Pr), up to 50 mg daily, *vit B12*, (Pr), up to 50mcg daily (or injections); *vit B15* (increases efficiency of oxygen handling), from 50 to 150mg daily; folic acid, (Pr), up to 50mcg daily; *biotin*, up to 300mcg, three times daily; niacin; *vit C*, up to 10g daily (some very ill people use even more; large amounts may be given intravenously); *calcium pantothenate*, 500mg daily (taken at a different time from elemental magnesium), up to 400mg in divided doses or near meals; *vit D*, (Pr), 400 IUs daily; *vit E*, 20 IUs daily.

Supplements for endocrine support *Thymus gland supplements*, along with the *amino acids L-ornithine and L-taurine*, plus extracts of *adrenal, pancreas and spleen glandulars* are a basic endocrine support. *Thyroid glandular, iodine or seaweed extract* may be used as well.

Supplements *Garlic, Fresh, Kyolic, and Pure-Gar deodorised garlic* *powder.* Garlic is high in minerals, vitamins and germanium.

These suggestions are drawn from recommendations made by New Zealand holistic practitioners; *Nutritional Medicine,* by Dr Stephen Davies and Dr Alan Stewart, Pan, 1987; and the writings of Drs William Crook, Leon Chaitow, William Philpott, Lendon Smith, Robert Erdmann and Orian Truss.

BOOKS TO READ:
Nutritional Medicine, by S. Davies and A. Stewart, Pan, 1987.
The Yeast Connection, by W.M. Crook, Professional Books, Tennessee, 1984.
The Yeast Syndrome, by J.P. Trowbridge and M. Walker, Bantam, 1986.
Health on your Plate, by J. Pleshette, Arrow, 1983.
The Amino Revolution, by R. Erdmann and M. Jones, Century Hutchinson, 1987.

PAIN RELIEF
Candida and hidden allergies are important and often unsuspected causes of chronic pain. Steps should be taken to correct both.
Magnetic therapy As outlined by Dr W.M. Philpott, this may provide relief with no known side effects.
Tricyclic antidepressants: Prothiaden and Sinequan in particular have been found helpful, perhaps by their effects on neurotransmitters in the brain.
DLPA, DL-phenylalanine An essential amino acid, inhibits enzymes which destroy the body's pain-killing hormones. Completely safe and non-toxic. Start with two 375mg tablets 15-30 minutes before each meal (for a total of six tablets daily), and continue until a substantial degree of pain relief is experienced; in some cases, as long as 2-3 weeks are required. If no relief is seen after 3 weeks, double the dosage for another 2-3 weeks. When relief occurs, reduce dosage gradually, step by step. (Should not be used by phenylketonurics or in conjunction with MAO inhibitors.)
Correction of acid/alkali imbalance Systemic acidity is a possible and unsuspected factor in much chronic pain. A visit to a well-qualified naturopath may be helpful.
White willow bark capsules as prescribed by a naturopath.
Acupuncture, chiropractic, osteopathy, massage, electroneurolo-

gical stimulation (TENS), neurolinguistic programming, rebirthing, biofeedback, visualisation and meditation can all be helpful.

BOOKS TO READ:
The Challenge of Pain, by R. Melzack and P. Wall, Penguin, 1982.
New Hope, by Dr. W.H. Philpott, 1987.
DLPA – the Natural Pain Killer and Anti-depressant, by Dr A. Fox, Thorsons.

TONIFICATION AND ENERGISATION

Acupuncture An energiser, tonifying organs, and balancing body systems. This is usually helpful, though some people have been known to react badly. It is not known whether their experiences were due to poor techniques on the part of their acupuncturist, or whether acupuncture unsettled their body's equilibrium to such an extent that disorder followed. The appropriate Chinese tonifying herbs reinforce the benefits of acupuncture.

Magnetic therapy Medical magnets used under direction often result in a general tonification of the system.

Ephedrine An old fashioned asthma remedy which increases the flow of oxygen around the body, relaxes bronchial muscles and slightly raises blood pressure. Can be used in herbal form (ephedra) as in Brigham tea, or by prescription. Some people benefit greatly, others find it less helpful. Use with caution. 1/4 tablet Pseudoephedrine (Sudomyl) taken twice daily on a full stomach may be helpful for bladder problems. Should not be taken in conjunction with monoamine oxidase inhibitor anti-depressant drugs. Derived from the herb Ephedra.

Adrenal extract Energises by strengthening adrenal gland function and adrenalin levels.

Organic germanium – germanium sesquioxide Some have found this helpful.

Guarana A South American herb with an energising effect.

TINNITUS

Tinnitus, or noises in the ears, often follows viral infections. Unsuspected middle ear disease may be a common cause of giddiness, vertigo, unsteadiness when walking and nausea. Specific treatment aimed at removing viral or bacterial residues and in-flammation of the middle ear may result in an overall improvement of the patient's condition. Increased fluid intake is sometimes helpful; or reducing salt intake. A few are helped when salt intake is increased. Chelation therapy, removing mercury amalgam, medical magnets and eliminating candida overgrowth have all been found helpful.

Zinc supplementation If buzzing or drumming in the ears is accompanied by fragile fingernails and thinning hair, zinc supple-ments may be helpful for all three. Homoeopathic zinc has also been found effective.

Anti-histamines Worth trying for symptoms resembling those of motion sickness. Scopalmine patches placed on the skin behind the ears may help if symptoms are similar to motion sickness. They have marked side effects for some people.

VIRUSES – ANTI-VIRAL AGENTS

Note that anti-viral drugs are all very new; extremely expensive; not always obtainable; not always helpful; often have severe side effects; need great skill in prescribing; and can only be a small part of the wider approach. Homoeopathic constitutional remedies and the new naturopathic oxygenating and revitalising preparations are helpful in strengthening the immune defence.

Echinacea Herbal tinctures are the most convenient way of taking this anti-viral herb: 20 or 30 drops every two waking hours for 10 days; then a week's maintenance regime of 7 or 8 drops a day; then return to the full regime. Also an immune-enhancer.

Homoeopathic preparations Constitutional remedies have been effective for some. Anti-viral preparations are more successful when used on a preventive basis.

Zovirax – Acyclovir (DA) Helpful in the treatment of herpesvir-uses. The cream for genital herpes; eye ointment for herpes simplex keratitis; orally for herpes simplex infection of the skin and mucous membranes; intravenously or by infusion for immunocomprised patients. Can have moderate side effects.

Ampligen (DA) A new therapeutic agent. A mismatched, double-stranded RNA molecule, it is effective against cancer cells. It is being used in AIDS and to treat brain lesions in both AIDS and CFS patients. Usually by transfusion once or twice a week. Few side effects.

Immunovir – inosine pranobex (DA) Enhances the immune response; used with AIDS. Expensive. Acceptable side effects.

Peptide T (DA) A natural brain hormone now being manufactured for therapeutic use against viruses that disable helper T cells.

Ribavirin This inhibits the enzyme reverse transcriptase found in retroviruses, and protects the body from further viral infection. Some consider it the most effective of all such inhibitors. Severe side effects for some.

BOOKS TO READ:

Living with AIDS – reaching out, by Tom O'Connor and Ahmed Gonzalez-Nunez, Corwin Publishers, San Francisco, 1987.

Psychoimmunity and the Healing Process: a holistic approach to immunity and AIDS, Jason Serinus, ed., Celestial Arts, Berkeley, California, 1986.

ESSENTIAL NUTRITIONAL

APPROACHES

Unless the doctors of today become the dietitians of tomorrow, then the dietitians of today
will become the doctors of tomorrow.
ALEXIS CARREL, *Man the Unknown*, 1935.

Removing the overload of those foods which are hidden factors in
an individual's illhealth is a major step forward, even for people so
sick that they think their case is hopeless. Detection and avoidance
of problem foods are usually done through a specialised dietary
approach:

1. An Elimination Diet – which removes all food allergen residues
from the body over a period of 5-7 days, and creates a degree of
sensitivity. Questionable foods are reintroduced, and detectable,
often immediate reactions occur with foods causing intolerances.
This is followed by:
2. A Rotational Diet – a long-term eating plan which allows the
body to heal itself. It ensures that the same foods (or foods from the
same food families) with their same chemical constituents, same
additives and contaminants are not eaten daily. This avoids any
build-up of potentially allergenic substances to a point where
symptoms occur.

The foods most likely to provoke intolerances – and therefore
reactions – are nearly always the ones most frequently eaten. For
people with immune dysfunction, the Western habit of eating only a
few different foods, day after day, is a recipe for disaster. For

example, eating Weetabix every breakfast and having sandwiches or hamburgers regularly for lunch may lead to wheat intolerance; daily eggs may lead to sensitivities to egg protein or chicken meat; coffee and tea with every meal may lead to caffeine addiction and intolerance; excessive sugar use daily (including regular snacks or fresh and dried fruits) may lead to sugar intolerance and addictive cravings; excessive milk or cheese may lead to an intolerance of dairy products.

Some foods have a bad track record for causing ongoing problems such as aching joints, headaches, oedema (puffy tissues), asthma and respiratory problems. Wheat, corn, eggs, chocolate, cow's milk, sugar and caffeine are special culprits. The hallowed tradition of a bottle of milk a day for children may need to be scrapped along with junk food. Clinical ecologists are firmly of the belief that cow's milk is primarily for calves, not for human beings, and that the dairy industry benefits most from the human ingestion of milk. Children with allergic tendencies who drink cow's milk are far more likely to go on to develop runny and stuffy noses, glue ear, sinusitis and digestive problems.

Both the elimination and rotational diets described here owe much to the insights of Dr Richard Mackarness who believes that the human digestive system and metabolic processes have not evolved quickly enough to keep up with recent changes in human diet. Human beings ate very much the same foods for hundreds of thousands of years ... roots, meat, fish, fruit, nuts, mixed wild grains and herbs. Concentration on single grains, such as wheat or rice, and the consumption of dairy foods have occurred only in the last 10,000 years as mankind settled down and became farmers. During only the last 100 years, mass markets have arisen and pre-cooked canned and frozen foods, refined carbohydrates, sugar and food additives have become major features in the Western diet.

Thus the basic diet to avoid food sensitivity is composed of the foods that mankind has eaten down through the centuries. It is low in grains and dairy foods, moderate in fish and meat, and high in vegetables, herbs, nuts and fruit. It avoids processed and packaged foods completely. Moreover, it reflects climatic and ethnic differences. For people of Polynesian ancestry, the most suitable Stone Age Diet will be high in fish, taro, kumara, birds, coconut, eels, breadfruit. Those whose forebears came from Scotland should emphasise apples, oats, barley, cabbage, red meats and fish. The English need a higher proportion of salad vegetables and a wider fruit choice . . . and so on. Thus, individuals selecting foods for the basis of their elimination diet would do well to consider the nutrition of their ancestors. These choices will also provide a useful basis for life-long nutritional regimes.

Following the rotational regime needed to remove the overload of circulating proteins and chemical substances arising from food allergens requires honesty and 'stickability'. Honesty – because there is no way that dieters who cheat can fool their bodies. 'Stickability' – because the regime must be followed to the letter, often for several months. But the end result justifies the pain. Once the immune system and the body's tissues have healed, a wider food choice awaits the strong-minded.

Whatever dietary approach is used, it should fulfil the following:
- Purifying the body so that it is possible to discover reaction-causing food;
- Eliminating all possible culprit foods from the body, and challenge-testing – introducing them one at a time;
- Eating fresh, freshly-prepared organic foods – avoiding chemicals, artificial flavourings, additives, sugar and refined carbohydrates which can increase allergic reactions, affect enzyme and hormone functioning, feed yeast growths and contribute to immune overload;
- Supplying proteins, carbohydrates, minerals, vitamins, amino acids and essential fatty acids necessary for health and immune restoration);
- Supplying special nutrients for body systems or organs being targeted by the disease process, e.g. the brain and nervous system, endocrine glands, liver and spleen;
- Drinking sufficient liquid to thin the thicker CFS blood may be helpful – up to eight glasses of pure water daily;
- Balancing the intake to the ability of enzyme systems to metabolise particular foods – rotational eating.

Whatever the diet, thorough chewing of each mouthful is an important aid to digestion. Enzymes in the saliva help particularly in the digestion of starches. Aim for at least 30 chews for every mouthful, specially when eating raw foods.

The information given in this chapter is but a brief guide to helpful dietetic approaches to reducing the burden of culprit foods and indicating sound nutritional principles. Because each person's metabolism is unique, and nutritional requirements alter as health is regained, individually tailored diets are necessary. Experimentation is often needed. Any person considering food avoidance should discuss the matter with a health professional before embarking on what can often be a complicated and even risky process. No matter the approach used, it should be carried out under the guidance of someone with experience. Ways of tracking down culprit foods, other than elimination dieting, are described in Chapters 12 and 14. Again, they should be attempted only with the support and guidance of a health professional.

ELIMINATION DIETS TO DETECT FOOD INTOLERANCES

The simplest method of tracking down foods and substances causing reactions is to eliminate suspect foods from the diet for at least five days and up to two weeks. This can be carried out by fasting, or the five to seven-day Elimination (or Exclusion) Diet and Challenge. The latter, which is the least traumatic approach, is based on Stone Age food. (See Appendix IV for full details.) Very highly allergic people may need to go on to the lamb and pears diet. This consists of roasted, grilled or casseroled lamb (including kidneys, liver and sweetbreads), peeled fresh pears, and bottled water. An alternative to lamb is turkey and turkey livers. Neither of these is recommended for people with heart disease or diabetes. All should be carried out only under medical supervision. A period of five to seven days is sufficient for the body to cleanse itself thoroughly of all reactive molecules. Only then should foods be introduced as outlined below.

A major drawback to the fasting and the very limited food choice is that it may unmask so many food intolerances that the unfortunate person may slip into the category of universal reactor and may end by finding there is almost nothing that is safe to eat.

With challenge testing, only one excluded food should be reintroduced on any one day. Have a good big helping at lunch or at least two cups or glasses of any liquid. Nothing else should be taken. People with extreme intolerances should introduce low risk foods, such as fruit and vegetables, before high risk foods such as wheat and dairy products. If there are any fixed allergies, those foods should be avoided permanently.

The pulse test, which is widely used as a back-up diagnostic tool in conjunction with food challenges, picks up immediate reactions. Before testing pulse changes, first establish the normal pulse rate by taking it several times during the day. Find the pulse spot on the wrist and count the beats for a full minute. Then take it again before trying a particular food. Take it again 20 minutes after eating; again, 20 minutes later; and finally, another 20 minutes later. A pulse change of 10 or more beats either way a minute is a strong indication of a food sensitivity.

Should a reaction occur, leave five days, or until the reaction has completely vanished, before re-testing the same food, and two to three days before introducing the next food. For delayed reactions, return to basic diet for more than two days or until feeling well again. Keep a food and symptoms diary, and record each food as it is introduced and any symptoms which they may cause. A page from Monica's diary is included as a guide. Reactions will vary from individual to individual.

Day 1-5: basic elimination diet. Pulse rate: 65-70.

Day 6: potatoes. Pulse rate: 68.

Day 7: soft-boiled eggs. Reaction: flu-like feelings, headache. Pulse rate: 85.

Day 8: basic elimination diet. Pulse rate: 68-70.

Day 9: basic elimination diet. Pulse rate: 68-70.

Day 10: wholegrain wholemeal bread. Pulse rate: 72.

Day 11: cow's milk. Pulse rate: 74.

Day 12: unboiled tap water (for chlorine and fluorine reactions, etc). Pulse rate: 72.

Day 13: sweet corn. Pulse rate: 68.

Day 14: sugar. Reaction: dizziness which lasted all afternoon. Pulse rate: 93.

Day 15: basic elimination diet. Pulse rate: 70-75.

Day 16: basic elimination diet. Pulse rate: 68-72.

Day 17: orange. Reaction: orange-red rash over upper body, tingling sensation. Rash lasted 30 minutes. Pulse rate: 86.

Delayed reactions occur most frequently after eating grains, making it difficult without the pulse test to pinpoint offending foods. Delayed reactions usually occur in a fairly predictable order, which helps to relate them back to the causative agent:

- Heartburn, indigestion and wind within half an hour of eating the offending food.
- Headache and mental symptoms within an hour.
- Asthma and rhinitis in an hour.
- Bloating stomach and diarrhoea within three hours.
- Hives and rashes within 6-12 hours.
- A noticeable weight gain due to water retention in 12-15 hours.
- Mouth ulcers, aching joints, muscles or back within 2-4 days.[1]
For ways to turn off severe reactions, see pp 149-51.

If there is no change in the level of symptoms at the end of the elimination diet, there are three possibilities:

1. The exclusion has been incomplete and a food is being eaten which causes reactions.
2. There may be sensitivities to chemicals and pesticides in the foods.
3 The problem is not caused by food sensitivities.

Following the detection of reaction-causing foods, the rotational diet should be followed:

ROTATIONAL DIET
The rotational principle is usually:

- a four-day rotation for the same food or a seven or 10-day plan for very sensitive people.

This provides for a diversified diet on a four-day basis for moderately allergic people, or a longer basis for those who are highly allergic. Unless the person is a multiple reactor, the diet plan should allow for a reasonable range of foods while building up ability to reintroduce the problem foods.

The permitted foods should be checked off against the food families guide (see recommended reading), and included in a diet plan which allows foods from the same food families to be eaten no more frequently than once every four days. Those adversely affected by one member of a food family may have trouble with another. This can be established only by trial and error.

The first day's menu might include peaches, avocado and lamb; the second papaya, lettuce, chicken; the third, grapefruit, beef and sweet potato; the fourth, pears, turkey and broccoli. The whole cycle might then be repeated. Foods causing reactions should be reintroduced only after there are signs of a definite return to health. If reactions are severe, see 'Allergies – treatment' in the preceding chapter.

Eventually it should be possible to return to even those foods which caused most trouble initially. Try to include them since they are often nutritionally valuable. If they cannot be rotated every four days, they should be tried once every eight days, or once every two weeks, or once a month. If they cannot be reinstated after three months, they should be tried again at six months or a year.

When reactions occur to a large range of foods, or when reactions are erratic and hard to interpret, then the effect of agricultural chemicals or additives should be suspected. This can be assessed by eating only organic foods.

People whose main problems are chemical residues and for whom reactions to food are not such a problem, should try a two-day rotation. This means that no items from any one food family should be eaten more than once every two days.

In order to prevent excess weight loss it may be necessary to introduce regular morning and afternoon snacks and supper into the diet.

Split-Day Diet The split-day minimum restricted four-day diet is a convenient rotational approach for people who are only mildly allergic. It starts the rotation day with the evening meal. It enables small helpings of 'safe' foods which have been eaten in the evening meal to be eaten also for breakfast and lunch the next day.

Eight-on-a-Plate Approach This is recommended for those having Enzyme Potentiated Desensitisation (EPD) injections. There may be more (or fewer) than eight foods; the aim is to eat small quantities of many different foods so that the body, strengthened by the EPD treatment, becomes habituated to them. A restaurant smorgasbord with many different dishes offers eight-on-a-plate. Asian dishes are usually more like 18-on-a-plate and, provided monosodium glutamate is excluded, are also suitable.

Amounts of each food range from one teaspoon to two tablespoons, preventing too much of any one food being eaten at once. This regime assists overall metabolism because it provides a wide range of vitamins, minerals, enzymes and other nutrients from

EIGHT-ON-A-PLATE DIET.

CHOOSE BREAKFAST, LUNCH, SUPPER AND SNACK MENUS IN THE FOLLOWING WAY....

Choose one from each category when planning your plate of eight:—No tinned or processed foods.

TEASPOON SIZE PORTIONS for the person with poor digestion.

TABLESPOON SIZE PORTIONS for those with improved digestion.

ORGANIC PRODUCE AND MEATS WHERE POSSIBLE.

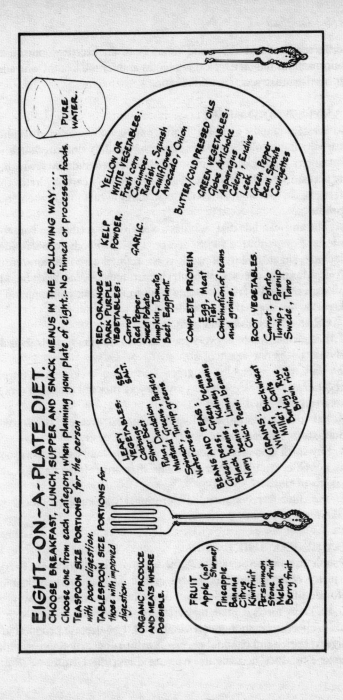

PURE WATER.

FRUIT
Apple (not Sturmer)
Pineapple
Banana
Citrus
Kiwifruit
Persimmon
Stone fruit
Melon
Berry fruit

SEA SALT.

LEAFY VEGETABLES:
Cabbage
Silver Beet
Ruha, Dandelion, Parsley
Mustard, Greens,
Spinach, Turnip greens
Watercress.

BEANS AND PEAS:
Green peas, Green beans
Black beans, Kidney beans
Navy, Chick Peas.
Lima beans

GRAINS: Buckwheat
Wheat, Oats
Millet, Rye
Barley, Brown rice

RED, ORANGE or DARK PURPLE VEGETABLES:
Carrot
Red Pepper
Sweet Potato
Pumpkin, Tomato,
Beet, Eggplant

COMPLETE PROTEIN
Egg, Meat
Fish
Combination of beans and grains.

ROOT VEGETABLES:
Carrot, Potato
Turnip, Parsnip
Swede, Taro

KELP POWDER.

GARLIC.

YELLOW OR WHITE VEGETABLES:
Fresh corn
Cucumber
Radish
Cauliflower, Squash
Avocado, Onion

BUTTER/COLD PRESSED OILS.

GREEN VEGETABLES:
Globe Artichoke
Asparagus
Celery, Endive
Leek
Green Pepper
Bean Sprouts
Courgettes

different foods at the same time. It is an excellent nutritional approach for the mildly food intolerant and for the healthy who wish to remain that way. (See illustration.)

ANTI-CANDIDA DIET

Western food, with its high content of sugar and refined carbohydrates, is ideal for yeast growth. Candida albicans flourishes on sugary foods and fast foods. To eliminate candida overgrowth, it is necessary to eliminate the sugars and refined carbohydrates that feed yeast, as well as foods containing yeast or fermentation products.

The anti-candida diet includes a wealth of vegetables and organic meats. For permitted foods, see pp 111-12. Foods to be avoided include: sugar, honey, brewer's yeast, refined carbohydrates, dried fruit, Marmite, cheeses, alcohol, vinegar, mushrooms, yeast breads, all canned foods, fast foods and junk foods. Fruit consumption is kept low or stopped for a while.

Other anti-candida diet guidelines:

1. Eat proper foods at every meal and do not miss meals. Snacks should be of raw vegetables.

2. Vary the vegetables – green leafy, root vegetables, purple vegetables, white vegetables. Vary the way they are prepared – raw, steamed, stir-fried, juiced.

3. Eat fresh meats only, preferably organically reared. Broil, bake, boil, steam or microwave rather than roast or fry.

4. Buy small amounts of meats and vegetables and eat them as soon as possible. Moulds grow on foods that are refrigerated for any length of time.

5. Individually recommended nutritional supplements should be taken according to advice.

DAIRY-FREE DIET

People can be sensitive to milk because of straightforward allergy, because of lactose intolerance, because of the many natural chemicals in milk, or because of the hormones and antibiotics given to cows. Dairy foods containing lactose are whole milk, skim milk, and some cheeses (including cottage cheese). Low lactose products are cream, butter and cheddar cheese. Yoghurt is also defined as a low lactose produce because the bacteria digest the lactose.

The world does not come to an end for those who have to avoid dairy products, just as it has not come to an end for the millions of Asian and Arab people who have little or no cow's milk in their diet, yet who live healthy lives with less bone deterioration than Westerners.

Vegetable juices, herb teas and pure water can replace milk. Fruit and carrot juices are not recommended, however, for those with candida. Dairy-free margarine and nut butters are a substitute for butter. Soy milk and icecreams are also available, and are delicious as well as being nutritious. Goat's milk may be acceptable to some, may upset others, and should be given to babies in small amounts only.

If there is concern about a low calcium intake because of dairy foods avoidance, all green vegetables, soybeans, parsley, bran, seaweeds, almonds and sesame seeds are good sources of calcium. The important thing is to eat vegetables, lots of vegetables, both raw and cooked.

RAW FOOD DIET

The raw food diet has been developed from worldwide research showing that uncooked vegetables and vegetable juices improve the health of the body's cells and increase resistance to illness. Raw foods contain a higher enzyme content which support the body's own enzyme systems. They also contain higher levels of minerals, vitamins, amino acids and fibre than do cooked foods.

Raw foods also help to cleanse the body of toxins and wastes which decrease energy and depress organ functioning. Fresh, organically grown raw foods contain many more nutrients, and even more 'living energy' than cooked or chemically treated produce.

The switch to a raw food diet should be carried out gradually, for instance by having a daily salad and adding fruits and vegetables until about 75 per cent of one's food is raw. Herb teas and fruit or vegetable juices should be drunk instead of tea or coffee. British writer Leslie Kenton has done most to promote raw foods and has written several books on the subject. Nevertheless not everyone is suited by this diet. Lightly cooked vegetables are often easier to digest.

GLUTEN-FREE DIET

Gluten is a protein found in several favourite grains, especially wheat. It is responsible for the stretchy, sticky nature of the dough. There are lesser amounts in oats, rye and barley.

If gluten is not avoided by those who are gluten-intolerant, a chain of illnesses may be set in motion. These include coeliac disease, irritable bowel syndrome and milder problems of the digestive tract. There is a genetic predisposition linking active hepatitis B with gluten sensitivity,[2] and anyone suffering the effects of hepatitis B should try avoiding gluten for a few weeks to see if there is an improvement in health.

People who are upset by wheat may actually have a gluten sensitivity and this distinction will need to be explored thoroughly. Nutritional supplements, particularly amino acids, are helpful in repairing the gut damage that is such a feature of this intolerance.

Non-gluten grains and sources of carbohydrates are: millet, corn, tapioca, amaranth, rice, pea and bean flours.

WHEAT-FREE DIET

Many people have reported major improvements in health, as well as loss of weight, simply by eliminating wheat from the diet. Wheat has the reputation of affecting the brain and emotions, and can be a background factor in alcohol addiction. Greater emotional stability, less irritability and clearer thinking are reported by wheat-sensitive people when they eliminate this pervasive grain from their diets. Its negative effects may be due to gluten sensitivity, fungal spores in the wheat, chemical residues, or repetitious eating of wheat leading to intolerance. Finding out which is a job for the expert.

A wheat-free diet seems almost impossible to Westerners used to having bread with everything. Scottish oatmeal porridge provides a solid basis on which to start the day. 'Think Asian' – and wheat and dairy products become irrelevant.

PRITIKIN DIET

Similar to the Stone Age Diet in that no processed foods or refined carbohydrates are allowed. Animal protein intake (chicken, lean beef or lamb and white fish) is limited to 15 per cent of total amount eaten. Totally excluded are butter, margarine, oils, nuts, seeds, salt and caffeine.[3]

People who follow Pritikin say that allergies disappear naturally and that overall health is greatly improved.

HYPOGLYCAEMIA AND A CORRECTIVE DIET

There are three types of hypoglycaemia. One is the result of autoimmune damage to the pancreas, such as is associated with diabetes; another is the result of insulin-producing tumours; yet another is the reactive type of hypoglycaemia associated with metabolic disturbances.

Reactive hypoglycaemia results in reaction to too much refined carbohydrate and too many sugary foods, and too much caffeine from the tea, coffee, alcohol and soft drinks in the diet. It is made worse by smoking, by chronic stress, by food intolerances, nutritional deficiencies and missed meals; by an underactive or overactive thyroid and by side effects from drugs.

The main symptoms of hypoglycaemia are: allergic reactions, weakness, feeling faint, fast heart beat, anxiety, irritability, insomnia, hunger, mood swings, mental and emotional disturbances, migraine and headaches. These are all confusing symptoms because they are so similar to those caused by food intolerances and candida. Nevertheless, for those whose symptoms are caused by hypoglycaemia, it is necessary to deal with this particular cause to correct the symptoms. Following thorough testing for reactive blood sugar levels and a diagnosis of hypoglycaemia, this regime (suggested by Dr Stephen Davies) is recommended:

1. A total avoidance of refined carbohydrates.
2. A diet that is EITHER high in complex carbohydrates, whole grains and beans and organic vegetables, OR high in proteins, meat, fish and eggs, and low in complex carbohydrates.

Some people are suited by one; some by the other. If the high protein diet is chosen, some find that 100-250mg vitamin B6, along with lecithin and pantothenic acid (B5), helps to steady their metabolism.

3. Small frequent meals – especially with the high protein approach.
4. People with severe symptoms at night often benefit by taking 5-15ml of glycerine before going to bed.
5. Avoiding tea, coffee, alcohol, cigarette smoking.
6. Having plenty of rest; naps after lunch, and early bedtimes.

7. Physical exercise, which can control blood sugar levels dramatically.

8. Stress management with yoga, meditation and deep breathing exercises.

9. Nutritional supplementation as outlined in the preceding chapter.

10. Reducing exposure to environmental allergens as much as possible.

DIET FOR CHEMICALS INTOLERANCE

Intolerances to foods may not be to the foods themselves, but to the chemicals they contain. These chemicals may occur naturally or may be added during food processing. They build up in the body, and reactions occur when the individual's overload point is reached. At this 'threshold point', many intolerances may suddenly appear.

The chemical clans are many. They include amines, salicylates, nitrates, tartrazine, benzoates, glutamate, and phenols. Sensitivity to naturally occurring phenols is thought by some clinical ecologists to be the first step in the allergy process. Constituents of almost all foods, phenols are particularly high in cow's milk, and tomatoes and other members of the nightshade family. Other ecologists believe alcohol intolerance signifies the first step in the allergy process. Reactions may be to the many chemicals contained in alcoholic drinks.

Salicylate intolerance is widespread in Australia, and has been closely studied in that country. Salicylates are found in aspirin, Disprin, apples, soft drinks and many common foods (see chart). Leonie Pullinger, a Tasmanian pharmacist whose child's problem reactions forced her to look beyond the straightforward food intolerance solution, told her story in a Tasmanian Allergy Association's newsletter. She said: 'No theory on allergy that we had read in various books and medical journals seemed to fit his case. Allergy theories claim overexposure to a food will lead to an allergy to it. He would thrive on the same foods for months on end. Others that he had never had, or had been exposed to in breast milk, or via utero, he reacted to quite dramatically on his first exposure.'[4]

A visit to the allergy clinic at the Royal Prince Alfred Hospital in Sydney answered many of Mrs Pullinger's questions. Her son belonged to the small overlap of food-sensitive people who had a genuine food allergy (in his case, to milk), and he was also intolerant to chemicals (salicylates) in foods.

Mrs Pullinger found, as so many others have done, that eliminating all foods containing a particular chemical can make a person ultra-sensitive, so that any consumption of that chemical will produce more severe symptoms. Control is usually achieved by a simple reduction in the amount of foods containing the particular chemical. The eight-on-a-plate approach is highly suitable.

The salicylate chart, prepared by Ann Swain, dietitian at the Royal Prince Albert Hospital in Sydney, is a guide to food choice for salicylate-sensitive people. (See next page.)

Other food-associated chemicals causing problems are:

Amines Bananas, cheese, chocolate, avocados, tomatoes, mushrooms, roasted nuts, liver, meat extracts, dried and salted fish, broad beans, pork, vinegar, yeast spreads, beer, wine.

Monosodium glutamate Canned tomatoes and mushrooms, soy sauce, parmesan cheese, blue vein cheese, camembert cheese, Chinese foods, commercial savoury foods, canned and packet soups.

Preservatives include: Benzoates: cordials, fruit-based drinks, soft drinks, dehydrated vegetables, beer. Sulphur dioxide: fruit products, minced meat, dehydrated vegetables, wine, fruit juice, dried fruit, some commercial salads. Antioxidants: commercial fatty foods, margarines, processed oils. Nitrates: ham, bacon, corned beef, luncheon meats, some sausages. Propionates: bread and other food containing yeast.[5]

MACROBIOTIC DIET

Macrobiotics is more than a diet; it is a medical approach and a way of life that aims to balance the body by balancing foods according to one's bodily condition. It is based on the theories of complementary opposites, of yin and yang, of sodium and potassium, of acidity and alkalinity.

Macrobiotic eating centres on whole grains (principally brown rice), beans and lightly cooked vegetables. A small amount of fish is permitted. Seaweeds are eaten as vegetables and snacks. They are highly nutritious, and alkalinise the blood. The macrobiotic diet has been judged to be nutritionally adequate by a U.S. Government committee.

SALICYLATE LEVELS

Negligible	Low	Moderate	High	Very High

VEGETABLES

Negligible	Low	Moderate	High	Very High
potato (peeled)	green bean	broccoli	eggplant	tomato products
lettuce	red cabbage	sweet potato	watercress	gherkin
celery	brussels sprouts	parsnip	cucumber	endive
cabbage	mung bean sprout	mushroom	broadbean	champignon
bamboo shoot		carrot	alfalfa sprout	radish
swede	green pea	beetroot		olive
	leek	marrow		capsicum
dried beans	shallot	spinach		zucchini
dried peas	chive	onion		chicory
red lentils	choko	cauliflower		hot pepper
brown lentils		turnip		
		asparagus		
sweetcorn				
pumpkin				

FRUITS

Negligible	Low	Moderate	High	Very High
pear (peeled)	pawpaw	pear (with peel)	passionfruit	sultana (dried)
banana	apple: Golden Delicious	apple: Red Delicious	apples: Granny Smith	prune
	pomegranate	loquat	Jonathan	raisin (dried)
	cashews	custard-apple	grapefruit	currant (dried)
		persimmon	avocado	raspberry
		lemon	peach	redcurrant
		fig	mandarin	loganberry
		rhubarb	mulberry	blackcurrant
		mango	tangelo	date
		tamarillo	nectarine	cherry
		most nuts	watermelon	blueberry
			lychee	orange
			kiwifruit	boysenberry
			almonds	

Negligible	Low	Moderate	High	Very High
			water-chestnuts	guava
				blackberry
				cranberry
				apricot
				strawberry
Salicylates are also found in tea, coffee,				rockmelon
most alcoholic beverages, most herbs and				grape
spices, garlic, honey, licorice, mint				pineapple
flavours.				plum

Salicylate Content	Amount Usually Tolerated
Negligible...............................	Any amount
Low	Any amount
Moderate................................	1 to 3 serves per day
High	Half a serve per day
Very High	None
One serve – 1 half cup of the food	
The following amounts are equivalent:	One serve from the MODERATE group
	One half serve from the HIGH group
	One tenth to one twentieth serve from the VERY HIGH group

Salicylates can cause a wide range of symptoms. Eat on a rotating basis below symptom level.

Macrobiotic specialists can be over-dogmatic about the necessity for a high proportion of grains in the diet. This proportion may not agree with people with CFS. Nevertheless the concepts of macro-biotics are important, and many have been incorporated into nutritional therapies for immune dysfunction.

IMMUNE-ENHANCING DIET
A positive approach to strengthening immunity by promoting metabolic well-being and strong, healthy cell walls is based on an increased intake of natural, organic foods high in certain lipids or

essential fatty acids (EFAs) and amino acids. EFAs regulate many body processes from basic metabolism (particularly of calcium), brain functioning, circulation and healthy nerve functioning.[6] Healthier cells and cellular membranes means that the body will be more able to expel viruses and other pathogens. This is the basis for the therapies of Emanuel Revici and his followers, AIDS specialist Dr Russell Jaffe, Dr Robert Erdmann and growing numbers of nutritionally advanced doctors. Their approach incorporates many features of macrobiotics. The overall nutritional recommendations that follow are being used, often with real success, by sufferers from many chronic immune disorders, including CFS, AIDS and multiple sclerosis.

EFAs particularly recommended include the Omega-6 fatty acids, linoleic acid (found in vegetables and grains) and arachidonic acid (found in organ meats); and Omega-3 fatty acids (principally in wheat, beans and fish). They are a first step in the production of the important hormones known as prostaglandins, abnormalities of which are a recurring theme in CFS. Deficiencies cause platelet abnormalities, poor circulation, inflammatory reactions, loss of smooth muscle (e.g. liver) function, allergies and underactive T cells in the immune system. Prostaglandins are not stored, and are made throughout the body. Their action is brief, since they are quickly inactivated by enzymes. For these reasons, prostaglandin production must be continuous. EFA shortages mean prostaglandin shortages.

A diet rich in the following foods is likely to protect the body against viruses and degeneration by improving the health of the cell walls, boosting prostaglandin production, and thinning the blood. Foods causing reactions should be initially excluded. Wherever possible, foods should be organically grown.

Linolenic acid: spinach, green beans, kale, lettuce, parsley, green peppers, bean sprouts, linseed (e.g. in porridge) and linseed oil.

Linoleic acid: brown rice, barley, corn, rye, avocados, tofu, pumpkin and sunflower seeds, sesame seeds and oil, walnuts, Brazil nuts and peanuts.

Gammalinoleic acid: thought to be particularly important in the treatment of CFS, is highest in oil of evening primrose, oil of borage and in blackcurrant and gooseberry seeds.

Arachidonic acid: at least 250 gms (½ lb) of fresh liver a week;

kidneys, sweetbreads, and venison.

Cervonic acid: mackerel, trout, tuna, crab, salmon, lobster, cod roe, cod liver oil, haddock, herring.

For those who are really unwell, some naturopaths recommend – using the above diet framework – starting with a liquid diet for the first week, with fresh vegetable broths, lentil broths, hatcho miso broth, vegetable juices, herbal teas and spring water. Cooked fresh organic vegetables should be added the second week; and cooked grains and meat broths can be added the third week. Fish and organically grown meat can then be added gradually, always watching for reactions.

A fatty acid booster may be helpful for the underweight, or those who are taking few EFAs in other ways. These contain the Omega-3 and Omega-6 EFAs that are so essential for prostaglandin production. Tom O'Connor recommends up to a tablespoon of the following oils in a four-day rotation: cod-liver oil, edible linseed, evening primrose oil, olive oil and raw sesame or grapeseed oil. Because immune dysfunction is often associated with over-acid bodies and over-alkaline digestive systems, it is important to eat as much easily digested alkali-producing food as possible. These include vegetables, fruits, seeds, honey, herb and bancha tea, miso – and common salt.

Very real difficulties arise in changing one's eating habits, not the least of which is finding the willpower to avoid one's favourite foods. But the benefits in improved health, happiness and weight normalisation are so great that, no matter how sceptical one's doctor may be about diet, it is a step that the ill person must take, whether in consultation with him (or her) or with a more holistically-minded health professional.

RECOMMENDED READING
The Yeast Syndrome, by John P. Trowbridge and M. Walker, Bantam Books, 1986.
The Yeast Connection, by William Crook, Professional Books, Tennessee, 1984.
Introducing Macrobiotic Cooking, by Wendy Esko, Japan Publications Inc, 1978.
Raw Energy, by Leslie and Susannah Kenton, Century Publishing, 1984.

The Food Allergy Plan, by Dr Keith Mumby, Unwin, 1985.
Nutritional Medicine, by Stephen Davies and Dr Alan Stewart, Pan, 1987.

Chapter 13   NUTRITIONAL APPROACHES

1   Breneman, J.C., *Basics of Food Allergy*, Thomas Springfield, Ill, 1978.
2   Harsanyi, Z. and Hutton R., *Genetic Prophecy: Beyond the Double Helix*, Paladin, 1983, pp. 60 and 107.
3   Thorough coverage of the Pritikin approach can be found in *The Pritikin Programme of Diet and Exercise* by Nathan Pritikin, now in its twenty-first printing.
4   'Case History: how food allergy theories didn't work', in *Meeting-Place*, journal of ANZMES (N.Z.), 24 May 1986, supplement.
5   ibid.
6   Rudin, D.O. *The Omega-∈ Phenomenon: Nutritional Breakthrough of the 1980s.* Sidgwick & Jackson, 1988.

SELF-HELP AND PREVENTION

Honour your body, which is your representa-
tive in this universe. Its magnificence is no
accident. It is the framework through which
your works must come, through which the
spirit within the spirit speaks.

From the *Sacred Convenant* of the Sumari,
an early Mediterranean people.

Self-help with its many approaches is a vital part of the healing
process. As the factors contributing to the overload are detected
and removed, the need for professional help diminishes. In the
process the sick person will discover that the body is the best healer
of all.

The body has a very real message when it tells the chronic fatigue
sufferer that it is tired, deathly tired, aching and weak. It says that it
wants rest if it is to heal, for it is during sleep that damaged tissues
are healed. Some people find they need double their normal
amount of sleep – and they should take it. There is no point in
having a stiff upper lip about the tiredness of CFS because avoiding
sleep and rest periods simply makes matters worse. Accept the
body's message – go to bed.

Likewise, if the body says that it cannot stand exercise, it should
not be forced to exercise. Many individuals with CFS who were
formerly energetic and athletic find it hard to accept that, for a
while at least, their bodies are no longer under their command.
They remember their fitness, and want to exercise vigorously. One
word for them – **DON'T**. Those who have done so (frequently after
having been told they should pull themselves together and that
exercise will do them good) often find their symptoms worsen. This

is not their imagination. It is not hypochondria. The pain that often accompanies even gentle exercise is due to the abnormal build-up of lactic acid in the muscles and is similar to that experienced by marathon runners. In their case, the pain comes after 12 miles or so. For those with CFS, a walk around the block may be too much. Muscles have been known to take years to return to normal, so it may be some time before former levels of exercise can even be contemplated.

Taking regular amounts of the tri-salts mixture (see under Allergy Treatments in Chapter 12) is often helpful in neutralising acid swings and reducing pain. Dr Emanuel Revici, the New York specialist in immune restoration (see pp. 59-62), recommends that, following exercise, only vegetables should be eaten. Grains, meat, fish and eggs should be avoided for some hours.

When the body is ready for exercise, then is a moment for rejoicing for exercise has a beneficial effect in reducing depression and clearing the mind. It can even help people recover from allergic reactions. The increased oxygen intake, circulatory stimulation and challenge to heart and lungs have a generally positive effect on overall fitness and feelings of well-being. Triglyceride and cholesterol levels improve and 'happiness' hormones (naturally produced endorphins) in the brain increase.

How much exercise is a matter for individual judgement. Towards the end of Alison's illness (Chapter 9), as her chemical imbalances were corrected, gentle jazzercise proved beneficial. A year earlier, any exertion sent her into a state of collapse. Another sufferer comments on the benefits of yoga; another on how much she has been helped by Tai-Chi, a Chinese exercise system that subtly links mind and body. It is often useful to record symptoms following exercise to see if there is a general worsening of the condition or if there are any specific problems with food.

Ten minutes' exercise with deep breathing at least three times a week is generally recommended for those who can manage it, as is gentle yoga. Deep, slow and regular breathing has special value since it increases oxygen intake. Breaths should be taken in right down to one's stomach. Even such unthreatening exercise as gentle stretching, walking or bicycling to the shops can help to keep one's physical structure in shape. Care should be taken to ensure that exercise does not mean further exposure to allergens. Most people with yeast overgrowth find that chlorine upsets them. For them, and for those who are sensitive to chlorine, swimming (showering or bathing) in chlorinated water should be avoided. Likewise, people who are sensitive to petrochemicals should not jog on busy streets or where there are high levels of pollution in the air.

PERSONAL PROTECTION

This means making sure that no substances causing reactions come in contact with the skin, mucous membranes and hair. It may mean throwing out many petrochemical-based personal cosmetics and toiletries, synthetic clothing, particularly underwear, and turning to natural ingredients and fibres such as cotton, silk, linen or wool. Those who are ultra-sensitive should take special care with woollen fabrics, for reactions are being reported to unsuspected chemicals used in processing or in pest control on the living sheep.

Reactions arising from household substances and cosmetics are often hard to trace. Toiletries and cosmetics causing reactions usually contain petrochemicals or distant derivatives. Preparations containing lanoline from New Zealand sheep are suspect because of the pesticides they contain. There are very few restrictions in any country on the materials used in cosmetics and toiletries, and few cosmetic companies make a regular practice of listing all ingredients on cosmetics packaging. As a result the customer has to find out by trial and often painful error. The effect may be no more than swollen eyes in the case of reactions to facial creams. In the case of the 39 French infants killed by hexachlorophene in baby soap, there was no second chance. Likewise, few would have guessed that a well-known brand of scented shampoo would cause nightmares in salicylate-sensitive children. It took the perceptive insights of many parents and an open-minded researcher to establish the connection.

Most disposable paper products, from tissues to disposable nappies, may cause reactions or weaken fragile energies in those already sensitive. Dr Phyllis Saifer tells the story of the mother and daughter who experienced itching and inflammation in the perineal area. The cause was finally found to be scented, coloured toilet paper.

Skin care should include washing regularly with mild soap and warm water and using a moisturising lotion daily and a sunscreen if any time is spent in the sun (particularly between 10 a.m. and 3 p.m.)

Stimulating and cleansing the skin with a loofah prior to bathing or showering is a healthful practice that boosts circulation in the minute capillaries beneath its surface. Adding two cups of cider vinegar or Chlorox to a warm bath and soaking in it for 15-20 minutes is an aid to detoxification. A cold shower following a hot shower will further stimulate the skin and close the pores. The old Chinese practice of slapping the body all over before dressing is also stimulating for those who are strong enough to carry it out and accept the stimulation.

Some sensitive people have reactions to deodorants. For them, there are special natural deodorising preparations. Likewise, there are natural toothpastes, or plain salt or bicarbonate of soda may be used.

TAKING CARE WITH SEX

Those with immune dysfunction need to take care in sexual relationships since they can affect the health of their partners through intercourse. Nevertheless Dr Alan Levin, immunologist of San Francisco, says: 'A regular, monogamous sex life is one of the best possible treatments . . . enjoy it with someone you love as often as you can. It not only makes you feel better, but it's a great motivator to take the steps you should take to get back to health.'

As sexual activity is intimately connected with the expenditure of energy, people without energy tend to lack interest in sex. This may be among the least of their own personal concerns, but a severe problem for their partners. Patience and empathy, less tiring positions and timing intercourse to coincide with energy highs are all helpful. Sufferers might encourage their partners to masturbate.

Semen itself is an immune-depressant and every new sexual encounter leads to an exchange of foreign antigens and possibly damaged immune complexes. Condoms are recommended for those with candida and severe immune problems. Oral contraceptives should be avoided as they disrupt hormone balance, are often potent allergens, and certainly increase susceptibility to yeast overgrowth.

For a candida-oriented approach to sexual hygiene, the candida checklist on page 111 should be followed.

THE HOME

Two major sources of allergens in the home may have to be dealt with if people have persistent CFS symptoms. One is petrochemical-based synthetic substances which 'out-gas', giving off toxic fumes. Such substances include the glue that sticks rubber-backed carpets to the floor; formaldehydes used in furnishing materials, particle board and foam insulation; varnishes and solvents used in furniture and timber fittings; furnishings made of synthetic fabrics; and household cleaners. The other is mould. Mould spores act like fuel to the fire of candida and allergies. All damp patches, mildew and sources of leaks should be dealt with.

'Squeaky-cleanness' and good ventilation are crucial to the health of the immune-compromised. A house that is poorly ventilated and poorly cleaned will have an atmosphere that is like a soup – swimming with moulds, dust, dust mites and bacteria; chemical fumes and tobacco smoke; microscopic fragments of animal dander; and cooking fumes and steam. Keep the floors and curtains vacuumed regularly. Dust-collecting knick-knacks and mould-producing pot plants should be kept to a minimum.

During intemperate weather it is tempting to keep all windows closed. Since out-gases and moulds build up in tightly closed buildings, it is preferable to be a fresh-air fiend, even if it means putting on another layer of clothes. Unless the weather is very cold at night (which may upset those with sensitive respiratory tracts), it is also wise to sleep with an open window. An ioniser placed beside the bed if often beneficial for those with respiratory sensitivities. By producing negatively charged ions, ionisers cause dust and pollutants to settle rather than float around in the air. Sensitive people often sleep better as a result. Bedrooms can be insulated from the rest of the house by putting weather stripping round the door.

When buying furniture, furnishings and household goods, look for natural materials such as cotton, linen, rush, wood, glass, tiles, slate, brick and metals. Formica and most hard plastics are safe. Soft plastics (such as in vinyl upholstery) and polyurethane foam are unsuitable in the homes of people with allergies. Mattresses should be innersprung, with cotton or wool padding. Some very allergic people are using all-wool or horse-hair mattresses, or cotton futons. Waterbeds are suspect in cases of candida overgrowth and have also been found to out-gas as the water temperature rises.

Fumes from gas cookers and heaters and oil heating systems often upset sensitive people. In general, electricity is preferable. Cookers and stoves should be well vented since steam from cooking fosters mould build-up. Cooking utensils should be of stainless steel, cast-iron, glass or best quality enamel ware. Aluminium is not recommended now that aluminium sensitivities are becoming increasingly common.

Incandescent lighting is preferable to fluorescent lighting which is thought to have a subtly debilitating effect on those with damaged immunity. Some become depressed if light levels are low, and it is worthwhile increasing the wattage before resorting to anti-depressive medications. Incandescent bulbs which give a light similar to that of sunlight are recommended.

There is a mounting body of evidence to suggest that constant exposure to unnatural electromagnetic radiation such as from overhead power cables, television sets, microwaves, home computers and cordless telephones affects cellular integrity and enzyme action. Cancer rates are higher for both adults and children living in the proximity of overhead power cables, or nuclear plants in those countries which have them. If there is particular concern, it may be possible to find a specialist electrical engineer to check electromagnetic levels and suggest corrective measures.

THE WORKPLACE

The 'sick building syndrome' is no catch-phrase. Heavy use of plastic and synthetic materials, fixed windows, electronic equipment generating ozone and other fumes as well as microwaves and microvibrations, newsprint, colleagues who smoke or use perfume ... these can all spell trouble for the sensitive person.

Those in problem buildings, particularly if the outside atmosphere is polluted or there are problem colleagues, should try for desks near windows in offices as high up as possible. They should keep signs on their desks that smoking is not welcome and should also press for smoke-free cafeterias and restrooms.

Those who work in factories or on sites where toxic fumes are present should forget about being macho or conforming to sloppy practices. They should insist on being supplied with masks; gloves if they are handling chemicals; good strong overalls and boots. Outer gear should be washed frequently – every day if contamination is high. They should check whether ventilation is sufficient and ensure that chemicals and fumes in the atmosphere are monitored regularly. Contact should be made with the Labour Department, union health and safety officers or public health inspectors should any employer pay insufficient attention to maintaining a well-ventilated and safe workplace.

Those who are working with electronic equipment such as computers, or with chemicals, should ensure they have fresh air breaks every two hours or so. The reasons should be explained carefully to employers, since many are unaware of the effects such working conditions can have. Go outside – breathe deeply, change visual focus, look at the distance. Shake your body around – and relax. If you wear glasses, take them off and let the sun shine on your eyes.

WATER

Chlorine, fluoride, various toxic chemicals and heavy metals traces are unsuspected causes of illhealth and neurological damage. High levels of bacteria or nitrates are dangerous for those with weakened immunity. Every effort should be made to find a good source of pure, uncontaminated water. If this is not possible, either bottled water or the purchase of a top quality water filter may be necessary.

As water quality deteriorates, local authorities usually increase the input of chlorine. One result is chlorine gas build-up in bathrooms, particularly during long hot showers. In New Zealand, over-chlorinated water resulted in the collapse of two elderly American tourists after they flushed adjoining toilets in a Southland motel. Where water is chlorinated, sensitive people should shower with windows open or extractor fans in operation. Swimming in chlorinated water is not advised either for the chemically sensitive or for those with candida.

THE GARDEN

Increased environmental consciousness invariably develops as sufferers realise the role of industrial and agricultural chemicals in illhealth of the globe and all living things. This often motivates those who have experienced CFS to join environmental groups, to search out organic produce and take up organic gardening. This is one very positive and practical way to take control of one's immediate environment and to protect health further by growing chemical-free fruits and vegetables. It has another advantage, in that even one small organic garden is doing a kindness to the earth.

The delight of growing healthy vegetables is secondary only to the joy of working with the earth, to seeing worms flourish and soil regain its vitality in the absence of chemicals. Even more joyful is the pleasure of working in the sun and natural light, of becoming aware of the elements and understanding the phases of the moon and their effect on growing things.

Organisations such as the Henry Doubleday Research Organisation and the Soil Association provide information about organics, with local meetings where members discuss gardening matters and hear speakers on related topics.

ALTERNATIVE TESTS FOR TOXIC FACTORS

The work of U.S. psychiatrist and behavioural kinesiologist Dr John Diamond offers people with AIDS, allergies and the chronic fatigue syndrome a pathway to health restoration and maintenance.

Behavioural kinesiology is based on the way that muscles weaken or strengthen according to the individual immune responses on exposure to various factors. Dr Diamond demonstrates the effects of food, art, music, poetry, facial expressions, posture, good news and bad in his book, *Your Body Doesn't Lie*. He found that many of the factors that weaken muscle strength are products of modern technology: refined foods, chemical additives and pollutants, drugs, hard rock music and synthetic materials. He confirmed the importance of the thymus gland (crucial in the production of T lymphocytes) in relation to the body's energy supplies.

The ability of various large muscles to resist pressure is thought to relate to energy levels in body organs and along meridians. A weakness in a muscle usually means there is a problem at the energy level in the associated organ. Various foods and nutritional supplements either add or detract from the body's energies. Energy-giving exposures will result in muscles testing strong and organs becoming strengthened. Energy-draining exposures have a negative effect on the body so that muscles and organs will test weak.

Muscle testing is widely used by naturopaths and holistic chiropractors as well as some doctors. It can be used for many applications but has one drawback. Another person is needed to carry out the tests, unlike the pendulum which is ideal for personal use, and will determine very much the same factors.

Both muscle testing and pendulum testing are helpful guides to choices of foods and dosage levels of nutritional supplements. They enable individuals to assume more responsibility for their health along with the confidence to try a wider variety of foods and have more flexible diets.

The pendulum is any small well-balanced object attached to a short length of string, metal or leather. It is primed when the person who wishes to carry out the tests holds it in his hand. This is thought to imprint it with the electromagnetic resonances of the body. It is then held over the object to be tested and allowed to swing naturally. Clockwise swinging means that the food is compatible with the metabolism of the holder at that time; anti-clockwise swinging means that it would be unwise to eat that particular food at this present moment. Backwards and forward swinging usually means 'Caution'. For a very few people, clockwise and anti-clockwise have the reverse meanings.

Germaine (Chapter 10) is one of those who was helped by the pendulum. It told her when she could safely add small helpings of steamed fish, chicken, and tiny amounts of root vegetables and rice to her green vegetable diet. It gave a good indication of how much medication she needed, and when. After Dr Y recognised her skill with it, his nutritional and medicational instructions included the words 'as per pendulum'.

'I had to learn and understand its workings, but the pendulum made all the difference in the world to my life. Sometimes things went amok, and I think it was because my mind was stronger than my body. Sometimes it seemed not to prevent me from overloading my body – but more often than not, it was accurate,' Germaine commented.

One remarkable example of the pendulum's sensitivity occurred shortly after she began using it. It gave consistently negative response to asparagus tips, but a positive response to the stalks. Using a Vega machine, Dr Y retested the asparagus, with the same results. This left Germaine and Dr Y confused. The next day, however, the newsmedia reported a viral fungus affecting local asparagus and consequent heavy use of anti-fungal sprays by growers – sprays which affected mainly the asparagus tips.

Allergies and intolerances respond not only to medications, various types of immunotherapy and avoidance, but also to techniques such as biofeedback, rebirthing, hypnosis and visualisation. These techniques aim to increase control of immune systems and harness individual healing powers. They have no side-effects, are easily available, can be practised at home, and are usually inexpensive. Albert Schweitzer said: 'Each patient carries his own doctor inside him. They come to us not knowing that truth. We are at our best when we give the doctor who resides within each patient a chance to go to work.'

The successes of mind-body practitioners such as Louise Hay, Stephanie and Carl Simonton, Bernie Siegel and Margo Adair in helping many people overcome supposedly fatal conditions such as AIDS and cancer, or prolong and improve the quality of their lives, make the healing of CFS appear a simple matter. Would that this were so. Not everyone has the ability to learn to influence subconscious processes, or the illness is intractable. Nevertheless, even if the steps forward are smaller, they will be steps forward.

The mind informs the immune system – and the immune system informs the mind. This is the message that people with immune dysfunction need to cherish. It is the pathway for information given by muscle testing and the pendulum. It is the basis for the many ways in which the chronically ill can put their own healing processes into action every day.

The following simple techniques are a first step towards gearing up the mind towards strengthening the immune response. They aim to link the brain with the inner self and with the myriad agents of the immune system. While they may be derided by some, they are practical, simple and scientific.

Sessions may last anywhere from five to ten minutes, or longer. Sit upright with spine erect, place your tongue over the top of your lower teeth, and touching the inside of your lower lip. Move gently into deep, full relaxed breathing, letting your stomach be the centre of your breathing. As you breathe, you will feel calmer, more centred and more aware of your breath as a source of energy.

Before you start, you might like to tap your collarbone (at the top of your chest, just under the soft portion of the neck) sharply several times. Thymus-tapping is practised by some people with AIDS, activating the body energies and actually stimulating the thymus.

You may experience tingling sensations in parts of your body, indicating that energy blocks are being opened.

Auto-suggestive affirmations can be used to calm mind and body before you turn your attention to specific matters. Imagine them as you say them, repeating each five times, while breathing slowly and steadily.

I feel calm and confident. My shoulders and neck (or anywhere that feels tense) are relaxed (relaxing each part in turn).

Specific affirmations might be:

Every breath gives me more energy. The oxygen I breathe in is bringing health to my fingers (or lungs, etc).

My immune system is awake, alert and effective. My blood is slipping through my veins faster – it is my greatest defence.

The (name of problem enzyme or enzyme system) is strengthening; it is becoming the perfect processor of (name of foods) within my body.

I have the power to make myself healthy – and this is what I am doing.

I am becoming healed in body, mind and soul.

I have a wonderful body and I love my body.

Everything that is good in the universe is protecting me.

DURING PREGNANCY

The best time to be concerned about the health of a child is prior to conception. American nutritionist Dr Jonathan Wright claims it takes four generations of optimum diet for full immune protection to be regained following one zinc-deficient pregnancy. The mother's health, and in particular her vitamin C and zinc status, are thought to be especially important to the health of her child.

Both parents need to take care with their diet, avoid smoking totally, and drinking to excess. Ideally speaking, oral contraceptives should be discontinued at least three months before conception. The mother-to-be should avoid stress, ensure that her diet is well-balanced and that she is well-supplied with vitamin C, zinc and iodine in particular. Reducing or even avoiding cow's milk completely is helpful to many pregnant women and to their babies. A diet rich in fresh vegetables (organic if possible) will supply a great deal of the needed calcium. Calcium supplements can also be taken if desired. This regime reduces the likelihood of future dairy product intolerances in children.

Zinc is a critically important element which must be available to the developing foetus in adequate amounts, for normal development. Zinc deficiency in the mother can alter the basic development of the child's immune system and some researchers conclude that adequate dietary zinc is essential during both pregnancy and lactation to ensure the development of an intact immune system in the offspring. Breast-feeding is even more vital in the development of immunity. The immature gut absorbs antibodies and many protective elements provided in breast milk.

Nausea and early morning sickness during pregnancy are both considered to signify nutritional, hormonal and other imbalances. Both conditions respond well to the dietary regime for hypoglycaemia or low blood sugar, which can be a real factor in feeling ill throughout pregnancy. It should be supported with this supplementation recommended by Foresight, the British Association for the Promotion of Pre-Conceptual Care:

Vit B6 – 50 mg once or twice a day; Vitamin C – 2000-3000 mg daily; Magnesium – 200-500 mg daily; Zinc – up to 50 mg daily (take at night, just before bed); Potassium 500-1000 mg daily; Manganese – 5-10 mg daily; Chromium GTF or chromic chloride – 200 mg daily.

CHILDREN

The general health of today's children shows alarming trends. Many babies are born with allergies and intolerances – almost unheard of only 40 years ago. There is an accompanying sharp rise is asthma, eczema, hyperactivity, learning difficulties and behaviour problems.

Many of these problems, which cause so much distress to all concerned, can be traced back to faulty metabolism, enzyme-related disorders and candida overgrowth. Eliminating milk and food colouring (therefore soft drinks, candies and icecream) from the diet of a hyperactive or troubled child may bring striking improvements.

Often children with constant infections and sore ears finish up by having tubes put in their ears to correct 'glue-ear', or they may have their tonsils and adenoids removed. The possibility of food intolerances should be fully explored before surgery is carried out. Dr

Crook recommends that those with 'glue ears' be taken off milk and given Nystatin and zinc.

Vaccinations and the threat of future viral illnesses are often in the minds of today's parents. With the spread of viral problems associated with CFS and the high incidence of illnesses following vaccinations, there is much to be said for building up the child's constitution as much as possible, and doing everything to strengthen its natural immunity. It may be helpful to consult a doctor who is also a homoeopath who will concentrate on the child's constitution and avoid the use of antibiotics.

Dr Cheney comments on the natural immunity to herpesviruses given by childhood chickenpox. As rubella (German measles) parties were once de rigueur for little girls, enabling them to catch what is in childhood a minor illness, he suggests that chickenpox parties for both boys and girls may help to avoid far worse illnesses in adulthood.

The fear of cot deaths, SIDS, is uppermost in the minds of many New Zealand parents in the light of their high incidence in this country. The following guidelines are suggested in caring for infants with possible salicylate sensitivity.[1] They relate to possible allergic reactions and withdrawal symptoms.

1. Artificial colour and flavours in foods and drinks and some fruits and vegetables with natural salicylates can affect a baby's breathing and increase the temperature if the baby is sensitive to these substances, and if considerable quantities of these foods are fed to the baby and then none at all. (For problem foods, see salicylate chart, p.186).

2. Caffeine (in tea, coffee and cola drinks) stimulates regular breathing. If a breast-feeding mother has a steady intake of caffeine, and then suddenly stops, the baby's breathing may develop long pauses (apnoea). The same occurs with alcohol.

3. For the first six months, babies should be breastfed, with no cow's milk supplements. The World Health Organisation recommends potatoes as the first weaning food. Other suitable weaning foods are cereals such as ground rice, mashed peas, lentils, fine ground meat and fish, bananas and peeled pears. Do not give artificial foods and juices.

4. Rinse clothing and bedding to leave no soap smell. Avoid shampoos, soaps and creams with perfume.

5. When putting the baby to bed, do not over-wrap or wrap too tightly. Ventilation and fresh air are important.

6. Do not expose the baby to cigarette smoke from anyone. Nicotine inhibits breathing and can pass to the baby through breast milk or from cigarettes smoked near the baby.

REACHING OUT

The most pertinent need for those with CFS is that holistically-oriented medical and health services are made available – and especially to those who cannot afford to pay for them. As the overload becomes heavier, as more infections become resistant to modern drugs, positive preventive health care is of crucial importance, not just to individuals but to nations. Any nation with sizeable numbers of its population laid low with chronic illnesses is a weakened nation.

CFS sufferers and their families will be in the vanguard of the growing army calling for change, a change back to natural methods and natural foods, back to the realisation their grandparents had of the importance of a healthy constitution and of 'right living'. They will:

• agitate for subsidies on nutritional supplements and treatments – both existing and those yet-to-be discovered.

• raise awareness of the need for good nutrition for pregnant women and nutritional supplements for young children.

• lobby for improved health education in schools and all institutions so that every school leaver is aware of the importance of good nutrition, hygiene and exercise.

• push for accessibility to methods of detecting and treating food intolerances, candidiasis, vitamin and trace element deficiencies, and the presence of toxic residues, with these to be taught in all medical schools.

• promote awareness of the need for holistic general practitioners who will specialise in 'regulatory homeostasis' – balancing immune, neurological and endocrine systems and treating accordingly.

• promote awareness of the need for special units where environmentally-sensitive and allergic people can be healed in surroundings that cause no reactive problems.

• argue for special programmes in prisons, psychiatric hospitals and institutions for the handicapped, to detect and eliminate allergies and chemical residues.

There is so much that those who are suffering from immune dysfunction syndromes can do to help themselves, their families and the wider society.

Overcoming the worst symptoms, so that a healthy anger can generate a determination that 'what has happened to me will not happen to others', will provide a springboard to positive action for the health of others and of the globe.

RECOMMENDED READING

Alternative diagnostic techniques:
Your Body Doesn't Lie, by John Diamond, Warner Books, 1979.
The Power of the Pendulum, by T.C. Lethbridge, Routledge & Kegan Paul (Arkana), 1984.
General detoxification methods:
Detox, by Phyllis Saifer and Merla Zellerbach, Ballantine Books, New York, 1984.
Mind and body:
Man's Search for Meaning, by Viktor E. Frankl, Washington Square Press, 1985.
You Can Heal Your Life, by Louise Hay, Hay House, 1987.
Love, Medicine and Miracles, by Bernie S. Siegal, Harper & Row, 1986.
Children and Family:
The Hyperactive Child and the Family: the complete what to do handbook, by John F. Taylor, Everest House, New York, 1980.
Why Your Child is Hyperactive, by B.F. Feingold, Random House, New York, 1974.
Chemical Children: how to protect your family from pollutants, by Drs Peter Mansfield and Jean Monro, Century Paperbacks, London, 1987. Particularly useful in identifying chemicals and grouping chemicals.
Breastfeeding Matters, by Maureen Minchin, Allen & Unwin, 1985.
A Good Start, by Louise Graham, Penguin, 1986.

Chapter 14   SELF-HELP AND PREVENTION

1   Holborow, P. Leaflet provided for allergy and hyperactivity groups.

15

GUARDIANS FOR THE EARTH

> We travel together, passengers on a little
> spaceship, dependent on its vulnerable sup-
> plies of air and salt; all committed for our
> safety to its security and peace, preserved from
> annihilation only by the care, the work, and I
> will say, the love, we give our fragile craft.
>
> ADLAI STEVENSON, 1965.

When asked why some people and not others develop chronic fatigue and immune dysfunction, New Zealand's Professor Campbell Murdoch said: 'They are our canaries ... the sensitive ones. Remember? The miners used to take them down the mines. If the canaries keeled over, it was time to get out.'

But we cannot leave the earth. This earth is all that we have.

Most human beings now live in a witches' brew of pollutants, pesticides and chemical additives to foods. 'The peoples of the modern world can be regarded as being engaged in a mass epidemiological experiment, which would never be approved by any government agency or committee,' says former scientific adviser to the U.S. Environmental Protection Agency, Dr Doug Seba. Yet the experiment, unplanned, unauthorised, unmonitored, continues on a scale so immense and with such unknown parameters that even the most informed find it hard to comprehend, and the most concerned do not know where to begin to take action.

Nature's systems are being buffeted and stretched beyond their threshold of stability. These are age-old systems with which the globe has maintained the precise conditions needed for all stages of the development of life. This regulation of the environment has continued for several billion years through complex feedback mechanisms based on chemical balance and biological life. But now the warnings are apparent in every country and every corner of the globe.

Worldwatch president Lester Brown believes the steps needed to restore the health of the globe have no precedent. 'Previous generations have always been concerned about the future, but ours is the first to be faced with decisions that will determine whether the earth our children will inherit will be habitable,' he said in 1987.

People look to governments for protection. Governments, after all, were originally formed to act in the interests of their citizens, to protect them against invaders, to provide a basis for prosperity and to establish codes of conduct enabling people to live without fear and in liberty within an agreed framework of behaviour. Yet in today's Alice-in-Wonderland world, many of the policies enacted by those elected to serve are contrary to the long-term interests of their peoples. Little protection is afforded against the excesses of industry and big business.

Changes in direction would seem obvious, yet the grip of technology and the status quo is so great that determined moves towards environmentally conscious, ecologically balanced societies offering quality of life are far more difficult to make than recognition of the problem would indicate.

In spite of the very real danger that chemical pollutants pose to the environment, it is still difficult for citizens to make headway against the big chemical companies. The latter have the finance to fight legal actions whereas the obstacles faced by individuals and citizens' groups in raising funds for legal battles put them at a further disadvantage. Those whose health has been damaged by environmental pollutants have to prove the connections. Whether they are residents' associations, national environmental groups, or children with leukaemia triggered by living near a nuclear power plant or by farms heavily sprayed with toxic chemicals, the onus of proof is on them, rather than on the offenders to prove their innocence.

Plaintiffs are further handicapped by lack of specialist knowledge and find it difficult to obtain up-to-date and accurate information. Governments are notably chary of handing out data on the ingredients of agricultural chemicals and the illhealth they cause.

A member of the New Zealand Pesticides Board, Margaret

Peace, is so alarmed at the generous use of pesticides that she took the unprecedented step in 1986 of issuing a challenge to cabinet members of government. Following a discussion of the illhealth of soil, stock and humans, she said:

'The chemical warfare on pests is never-ending and the only winners are the international chemical companies. The only final solution lies in applying ecological principles to crop production. Disease-prone and parasite-infected crops are signs of an ecosystem under stress, most significantly a soil artificially "fed" with inorganic fertilisers and lacking the micronutrients of a healthy natural organic soil.'

Yet all is not bad news. By 1988, 22 governments, including those of the United States, Great Britain, Mexico and New Zealand undertook to reduce the manufacture of chlorofluorocarbons in order to slow down the rate of damage to the ozone layer. Furthermore, the major United States' manufacturers and those in New Zealand have gone further than the international agreements by voluntarily speeding the phase-out of CFC's.

Right-to-know laws in the United States, described by environmentalists as 'an idea whose time has come', give everyone the right to know what toxic chemicals they are exposed to. If local authorities spray along the fence line, or farmers spray across the valley, people have the right to know what is being sprayed. They also have the right to protest. Workers have the right to know what is in any chemical mixture they work with, and what it is likely to do to them.

The United States Supreme Court recently ruled that all emission rates in the United States must be based solely on health grounds. In the past there were many excuses. Now industries have to comply, or they have to shut down. Also in 1988 the Environmental Protection Agency finally served notice on 14 metropolitan areas that no new major industries would be permitted until pollution levels dropped.

Enormous challenges lie ahead. The first that must be met is a drastic reduction in the use of those agricultural chemicals which harm or destroy life, along with a return to predominantly organic farming. Its success rests on determination and an informed attention to the health of ecological systems and the state of the soil so that its vitality can be built up through all possible biological means. This is very far from simple. It may mean a switch from the capital-intensive type of farming which relies on chemicals for productivity to labour-intensive farming such as was carried out for several thousand years prior to World War II. It means re-educating farmers brought up to spray and drench with poisonous chemicals, and educating the many new workers who would be required to help work the land. It means reafforestation, especially on marginal lands, with farming confined to the better soils. It might mean a new approach to farm ownership and profitability with follow-on effects on the entire economic structure.

The next challenge is the re-ordering of transport. The use of petroleum products is a major cause of air pollution and a major factor in both acid rain and the destruction of the protective ozone layer. The technology is here at this minute for a switch from petroleum fuels to methanol and ethanol and for emission reduction in coal and oil burning plants. The development of both hydrogen fuel cells for electric-powered vehicles and hydrogen-burning technology is already far advanced. What is needed is determination on the part of governments and acceptance by the oil and energy companies that the welfare of the world and its people takes precedence over everything else. Extremely strict chemicals policies, well-funded chemicals inspection and draconian punishments for offenders are essential. Perhaps most important of all are public education and the kindling of a determination for change.

The 'canaries' described by Professor Murdoch will be in the vanguard of those pushing for changes to protect all living things, and for a re-ordering of medical approaches and systems. They need not fear that theirs will be the only lonely voices in the wilderness. With every misspent year, they will be joined by many more, until the wilderness is filled with cries for change.

Among the many activities open to everyone, as self-elected guardians for the health of the earth and all living things, are:

Learning, reading, self-education.

Writing to elected representatives about pesticides, pollution and the causes of their own individual illhealth.

Raising the consciousness of others by speaking to individuals, to groups and to the media.

Becoming educators of receptive media people.

Drawing the attention of the media to chemical spills and

mismanagement.

Voting for environmentally-conscious candidates in elections.

Supporting groups that are active in the earth's defence, such as Friends of the Earth, the Sierra Club, Greenpeace, Forest and Bird Society, Pesticide Action Network.

Giving information to their doctors on the causes and treatments of chronic fatigue and immune dysfunction.

Complaining to local authorities about spraying.

Complaining to supermarkets about food additives and chemically treated produce, and asking for organically produced foods.

Monitoring toxic chemicals in garden shops and supermarkets.

Investing only in environmentally sensitive companies.

Working to consolidate all that leads to health in their homes, their gardens, their farms, their communities and their nations.

Each individual effort to reduce the overload of pollution and to discover and nurture the links which tie all living things together has a positive effect, small though it may be.

It is still possible, indeed it must be possible, to restore the earth to health, although plainly this is the most exacting and complex undertaking ever to face human beings. Health for humanity is inseparable from health for the earth.

APPENDIX I

AN ILLNESS WITH MANY NAMES ...

These are some of the many names for the same or closely related manifestations of the Chronic Fatigue Syndrome – or Chronic Fatigue and Immune Dysfunction Syndrome.

Abortive poliomyelitis
Acute disseminated encephalomyelitis
Allergic tension fatigue syndrome
Allergic toxaemia
APICH syndrome (Autoimmune, Polyendocrinopathy, Immune disregulation, Candidosis, Hypersensitivity)
Atypical poliomyelitis
Acute infective encephalomyelitis
Akureyi disease (Iceland)
Benign myalgic encephalomyelitis
Benign subacute encephalomyelitis
Chemical hypersensitivity syndrome
Chronic brucellosis
Chronic candidiasis
Chronic Epstein-Barr Virus – CEBV
Chronic fatigue syndrome – CFS
Chronic fatigue and immune dysfunction syndrome – CFIDS
Chronic influenza (Italy)
Chronic mononucleosis syndrome
Chronic vital fatigue syndrome
Da Costa's Syndrome (American Civil War)
Damadian's Ache
Depression
Dreaded Lurgy (U.K.)
Dysfunction syndrome
Ecological illness
Effort syndrome (U.K.World War II)
Encephalitis lethargica

Encephalomyelitis – benign encephalomyelitis
Encephalomyelitis resembling poliomyelitis
Encephalo-neuro-myasthenia – E.N.M.
Encephalitis resembling poliomyelitis
Environmentally ill – E.I.
Epidemic malaise
Epidemic myaligic encephalomyelitis – EME
Epidemic vegetative neuritis
Epidemic diencephalomyelitis
Epidemic myalgic encephalomyelitis or encephalomyelopathy
Epidemic pseudoneurasthenia
Epidemic neuromyasthenia – E.N.M.
Epstein-Barr Virus syndrome
Fatigue sickness
Fibromyalgia
Fibromyalgie syndrome (esp. in Holland)
Fibrositis
Food and chemical sensitivity
Functional disease
Hidden allergies
Hollywood Blahs
Icelandic disease
Lymphocytic meningo-encephalitis
Lymphoreticular encephalomyelopathy
Maladaptation syndrome
Modern environment illness
Myalgic encephalomyelitis – M.E.
Mystery disease
Neuromyasthenia
Persistent myalgia following sore throat
Post-infection encephalomyelitis
Post-infection fatigue syndrome
Post-viral fatigue syndrome
Primary fibrositis syndrome
Psychoneurosis
Raphe nucleus encephalopathy
Ridgen's disease
Royal Free disease
Somatisation disorder
Spasmophilie (France)
Tapanui 'flu (N.Z.)
Total allergy syndrome

Twentieth Century Disease (U.S.)
Type 2 allergies
Unknown disease
Vilyuish encephalomyelitis (Siberia)
Yuppie Plague (U.S.)

APPENDIX II

RECORDED EPIDEMICS OR INCIDENCES OF CFS
(Under many names)

1934	Los Angeles	4.5% of hospital staff
1937-39	Switzerland	220 in military camps/ hospitals
1939	Harefield, England	student nurses
1948-49	Akureyri, Iceland	average 6.8% of popn in 3 towns
1949-51	Adelaide, Australia	1,036 cases, district epidemic
1950	Louisville, Kentucky	37 student nurses
1950	New York State	33 cases, district epidemic
1952-54	Denmark	70 cases, district epidemic
1952	Lakeland, Florida	27 cases, district epidemic
1952	Middlesex Hosp, London	14 student nurses
1953	Rockville, Maryland	50 student nurses
1953	Coventry, England	13 hospital staff
1954	Tallahassee, Florida	450 cases, district epidemic
1954	Berlin, W. Germany	7 soldiers on a military base*
1954	Seward, Alaska	175 cases, district epidemic
1954-55	Johannesburg, South Africa	14 cases, district epidemic
1955	Durban, South Africa	140 hospital staff
1955	Perth, Western Australia	district epidemic

1955	Boscombe, England	2 hospital staff
1955	Dalton, Cumbria, U.K.	233 cases, district epidemic
1955	Royal Free Hospital, London	292 hospital staff, 12 patients
1956	Newton-Le-Willows, Lancs	162 cases, district epidemic
1956	Iceland	not known
1957	Brighton, South Australia	60 cases, district epidemic
1965-66	Lamarque, Texas	not known
1970	Great Ormond St Hosp, U.K.	145 cases
1976	S.W. Ireland	100 cases, district epidemic
1976-77	Sydney, Australia	district epidemic
1977	Fort Worth, Texas	not known
1978	New Zealand	500+ in Otago province
1983-85	Tapanui, New Zealand	1000 cases in area, many cases throughout country
1984-86	Lake Tahoe, California	200 cases
1984	Gunnedah, N.S.W.	district epidemic, 300 cases
1985-86	Yerington, Nevada	100 cases
1986	Sydney, Aust.	170 cases Narabeen district
1988	New Zealand	very widespread; several thousands
1988	United Kingdom	widespread; est. 100,000 cases
1988	United States	widespread, cases in hundreds of thousands
1988	Australia	widespread, est. 10,000

APPENDIX III

A SYMPTOM CHECKLIST FOR CFS
Check if symptom is present:

1. _____ **Fatigue (95%), usually made worse by physical exercise**

2. _____ **Cognitive function problems (80%)**
   _____ a. Attention deficit disorder
   _____ b. Calculation difficulties
   _____ c. Memory disturbance
   _____ d. Spatial disorientation
   _____ e. Frequently saying the wrong word

3. _____ **Psychological Problems (80%)**
   _____ a. Depression
   _____ b. Anxiety, which may include panic attacks
   _____ c. Personality changes, usually a worsening of a previous mild tendency
   _____ d. Emotional liability (mood swings)
   _____ e. Psychosis (1%)

4. _____ **Other Nervous System Problems (75%)**
   _____ a. Sleep disturbance
   _____ b. Headaches
   _____ c. Changes in visual acuity
   _____ d. Seizures
   _____ e. Numb or tingling feelings
   _____ f. Disequilibrium
   _____ g. Lightheadedness, feeling 'spaced out'
   _____ h. Frequent unusual nightmares
   _____ i. Difficulty moving tongue to speak
   _____ j. Ringing in the ears
   _____ k. Paralysis
   _____ l. Severe muscular weakness
   _____ m. Blackouts
   _____ n. Intolerance of bright lights
   _____ o. Intolerance of alcohol
   _____ p. Alteration of taste, smell, hearing

5. ____ **Recurrent 'Flu-like Illnesses (75%) often with chronic sore throat**

6. ____ **Painful Lymph Nodes**, especially on the sides of the neck and under the arms (60%)

7. ____ **Severe Nasal and Other Allergies**, often a worsening of a previous mild problem (40%)

8. ____ **Weight Change**, usually gain (70%)

9. ____ **Muscle and Joint Aches** with tender 'trigger points', or fibromyalgia (65%)

10. ____ **Abdominal Pain, Diarrhoea, Nausea** – 'irritable bowel syndrome' (50%)

11. ____ **Low Grade Fevers**, or feeling hot often (70%)

12. ____ **Night Sweats (40%)**

13. ____ **Heart Palpitations (40%)**

14. ____ **Severe Premenstrual Syndrome** – PMS (70% of women)

15. ____ **Rash of Herpes Simplex or Shingles (20%)**

16. ____ **Uncomfortable or Frequent Urination**, pain in prostate (20%)

17. ____ **Other symptoms seen in less than 10% of patients**
    ____ a. Rashes
    ____ b. Hair loss
    ____ c. Impotence
    ____ d. Chest pain
    ____ e. Dry eyes and mouth
    ____ f. Cough
    ____ g. Temporo-mandibular-joint (TMJ) syndrome
    ____ h. Mitral valve prolapse
    ____ i. Frequent canker sores
    ____ j. Cold hands and feet
    ____ k. Serious rhythm disturbances of the heart
    ____ l. Carpal tunnel syndrome
    ____ m. Pyriform muscle syndrome causing sciatica
    ____ n. Thyroid inflammation
    ____ o. Various cancers (a rare occurrence)

Reprinted with permission of Jay A. Goldstein M.D.
9429 Beverlywood Street, West Los Angeles, CA 90034

Laboratory Tests for CFS as suggested by Dr A. L. Komaroff
These results are principally of interest to doctors.
Different tests are recommended in an ANZMES (NZ) information leaflet

Mild leukopenia (3000-50000/mm^3)
Moderate monocytosis (7%-15%)
Relative lymphocytosis (>40%)
Atypical lymphocytosis (1%-20%)
Slight elevation in SGOT and SGPT
Erythrocyte sedimentation rate unusually low (0-4mm)
Partial reduction in immunoglobulins
Circulating immune complexes (low levels)
Increased CD4/CD8 ratio
EBV antibodies
Viral capsid antigen – IgG > 1:640
Viral capsid antigens – IgM not detectable
Early antigen – Ab > 1:40
EB nuclear antigen – Ab   1:5

APPENDIX IV

THE BASIC DIET FOR FOOD SENSITIVITY

The following nutritional selection is the basis for foods in the Elimination Diet and in the Rotational Diet. Details of how to go about these diets are contained in Chapter 13, Essential Nutritional Approaches. During the elimination phase, all packaged, processed and manufactured foods should be avoided.

Setting up both diets requires planning and special shopping. Ideally, all banned foods should be removed from the house to reduce temptation. Put some time aside to prepare dishes in advance. They can be labelled and frozen for future convenience.

The initial elimination phase is a minimum of 5 days. Following that, foods from the 'Foods to Avoid' column should be introduced as outlined previously.

Breakfast is always the most difficult meal, since wheat, corn, eggs, and dairy products are not allowed. Try steamed vegetables, rice and fish or meat.

ELIMINATION DIET

ALLOWED	NOT ALLOWED
Meat	**Eggs**
Fresh or frozen lamb and beef, chicken.	Bacon, ham, corned beef, sausages or delicatessen meats.
Fish	
Fresh or frozen fish, also canned salmon and tuna (watch labels).	Crumbed battered fish, patties, fish fingers, fish in tomato sauce.
Fresh Vegetables (a) well washed	
Broccoli, spinach, cauliflower, cabbage, asparagus, brussel-sprouts, celery, bean sprouts, green beans, lettuce, red cabbage, green peas (fresh or home frozen), leeks, chives, swede, turnips, onions, garlic.	Tomato and any tomato products, gherkin, radish, capsicum, zucchini, peppers, cucumber, broadbean, alfalfa sprouts, watercress, mushrooms, egg plant, dried or frozen vegetables.

Fresh Vegetables (b) well washed
Potatoes, yams, kumara, beetroot, parsnip, carrot, marrow, pumpkin.

Soya beans and all soya products (unless told otherwise).

Fruit
Pears, washed and peeled.
Golden Delicious apples, washed and peeled.

Avocado, banana, other apples, all berries, stonefruit, grapes, currants, grapefruit, lemons, oranges, melons, prunes, raisins, passionfruit, rhubarb, pineapple, all dried fruit – dates, figs, etc.

Cereals
Brown rice, rice flour, Blackmore's puffed rice, rice wafers.
Arrowroot (for thickening), Millet, buckwheat

Wheat, oats, rye, barley, corn, semolina.

Drinks
Water.
Herb teas.

Decaff. coffee, tea, coffee, Milo, **milk**, soft drinks, fruit drinks, all alcoholic drinks.
No tobacco or marijuana.

Oil
Check label says COLD PRESSED OIL: Safflower.

Butter, dripping, Chefade, margarine.
Cheese.

Sweeteners
Nil.

Honey, sugar, malt, artificial sweeteners.

Condiments
Salt, pepper, sea salt, kelp.

Mayonnaise, any dressings, sauces, relishes, vinegar.

Medications
Check that all medications taken are known to the doctor. Panadol

All non-essential medications, including vitamins, minerals and

should be taken only if really
necessary.

herbs. Oil of wintergreen – Deep
Heat, Tiger Balm, etc.

Toiletries
Unperfumed deodorants.
Mix salt and soda, or just use salt
as a toothpaste.
Unscented, uncoloured
Neutrogena is acceptable for
personal use.
Sunlight soap or Amway 'Dish
Drops' and Laundry Liquid can
be used for dishes and clothes.

Aerosol products. Try to avoid
toothpastes, perfumes, talcum
powder, hair spray.
Check your make-up – it can
cause problems.

CONTACT ADDRESSES
SUPPORT AND ACTION GROUPS

Support groups proliferate as the need grows. In New Zealand alone there are more than 30 allergy awareness groups, with as yet no national link, and many local M.E. groups. Addresses of support groups, particularly at a local level, change frequently. Well-established societies, listed below, will direct enquiries.

U.K.
M.E. Association, P.O. Box 8, Stanford-le-Hope, Essex SS17 BEX.
M.E. Action Campaign, P.O. Box 1126, London W3 0RY.
Both the M.E. Association and the M.E. Action Campaign publish periodicals and other information for sufferers and supply addresses of local support groups. The M.E. Action Campaign also has available lists of knowledgeable and sympathetic doctors.
Action Against Allergy, 43 The Downs, London SW20.
Henry Doubleday Research Association, National Centre for Organic Gardening, Ryton-on-Dunsmore, Coventry CV8 3LG.
Greenpeace Ltd, 36 Graham Street, London N1.

Canada
Canadian Prolonged Viral Syndrome Association, 206-1172 Yates Street, Victoria B.C. V8V 3M8.

New Zealand
The Australian and New Zealand Myalgic Encephalomyelitis Society (Inc): ANZMES (N.Z.), Box 35-429, Browns Bay, Auckland 10. National organisation which has up-to-date addresses for regional M.E. support groups. Publishes the periodical *Meeting Place*, and other invaluable information on health problems related to CFS.
Christchurch M.E. Support Group, P.O. Box 29-143, Christchurch.
Auckland Allergy Awareness Association Inc. Box 12-701, Penrose.
Wellington Hyperactivity & Allergy Association, 93 Waipapa Road, Wellington 3.

Australia
M.E. Society, P.O. Box 645, Mona Vale, NSW 2103.
M.E. Society, P.O. Box 7, Moonee Ponds, VIC 3039.
Allergy Association Australia – New South Wales, P.O. Box 74, Sylvania,

Southgate, NSW 2224.
Australian Society for Environmental Medicine: Suite 4, Collins St., Melbourne, Vic 3000. Information service for doctors.

GLOSSARY

Acid base balance: a normal condition when the body makes acids and bases at the same rate they are removed.

Acid base metabolism: the processes that maintain the balance of acids and bases in the body. When this balance is upset, either too much acid is present (acidosis) or the opposite (alkalosis).

Acidosis: an abnormal increase in hydrogen in the body from too much acid or the loss of base. There are many forms of acidosis.

Addison's disease: a life-threatening autoimmune disease in which the adrenal gland is gradually destroyed.

Allergen: a substance that produces an immediate hypersensitivity reaction and the symptoms of allergy and asthma.

Allergy: an abnormal reaction on the part of the body to some foreign substance, which can be a food; exaggerated immune response to an allergen.

Amino acid: At least 22 are essential for life and must be included in the diet. 1. A group of atoms containing an amine group and a carboxyl group. 2. The building block of protein.

Anabolic: processes of construction and regeneration, of manufacturing new enzymes and protein structures.

Anergy: an immune defect in which the body does not fight off foreign substances well enough. As in advanced tuberculosis, AIDS, and other serious infections.

Antibody: a protein substance produced by B cells in response to an invading substance (antigen) – bacterial, viral, protein, fungal or chemical – and which helps destroy it.

Antigen: foreign substance that stimulates the immune response and the formation of antibodies. Antigens can cause allergic reactions.

Arginine: an amino acid essential to growth, strengthens immune system.

Arthralgia: aches and pains in one or many joints.

Arthritis: inflammation in a joint, with heat, swelling, pain and redness.

Atopic: a hereditary tendency to develop immediate allergies, such as asthma, allergic skin diseases or hayfever. Caused by antibodies in the skin or bloodstream.

Autoantibody: antibody directed against the body's own tissue.

Autoimmune: when the body's defences are turned against the body itself, leading to chronic and often deadly disease. Often switched on by virus infections which may retain the T cells to attack the wrong tissues.

Autonomic nervous system: part of the nervous system that regulates vital functions of the body that are not consciously controlled (involuntary).

B Cell: in the spleen or lymph nodes, replication is switched on by the helper T cells, produces antibodies against specific antigens. Produces memory cells which remember previous invaders.

Biotin: B vitamin essential to growth, present in every living cell.

Biotinidase: the enzyme that metabolises biotin: important in intestinal flora balance and candida control. Its functioning and levels are depressed by antibiotics. No natural deficiencies recorded prior to 1975; hereditary deficiencies now becoming relatively common.

Blood cells: Three main types are recognised: red blood cells (erythrocytes) which carry oxygen and carbon dioxide; white blood cells (leukocytes) help fight infection; platelets (thrombocytes) help prevent bleeding.

Candida albicans: a common yeast found in the mouth, digestive tract, vagina, and on the skin of healthy persons. If there is reduced immune competency, it may proliferate throughout the body causing widespread symptoms and chronic illhealth (candidiasis).

Catabolic: tears down existing protein structures, dismantles enzymes and hormones, and, in so doing, releases energy.

Catalyst: a substance or agent used to speed or maintain a reaction in which it does not participate; thus it may be used over and over.

Cell-mediated immunity: immune response generated by the T cells. Deficient with all the chronic immune-deficiency syndromes.

Cholesterol: fatty substance (EFA) made throughout the body from which steroid hormones are produced.

Clinical ecologist: a doctor who makes a special study of the way in which environmental factors and foods can make individuals ill.

CNS: central nervous system – the brain and the spinal cord – carries information to and from the peripheral nervous system. The main network of coordination and control for the whole body.

Collagen: the main structural protein of the body.

Collagen disease: diseases characterised by inflammation of connective tissues, especially the skin and joints – systematic lupus erythematosus, rheumatoid arthritis, etc.

Corticosteroid: hormones naturally made in the adrenal cortex; influence or control key functions of the body – making carbohydrates and proteins, workings and functions of heart, muscles, kidneys and other organs. Released during stress. Too much of these hormones are linked to autoimmune conditions and can cause severe side effects.

DNA: deoxyribonucleic acid, the basic genetic molecule and protein factory of the body; the only substance that can reproduce itself and the basis of life's processes. Lack of DNA production has profound effects on aging and degenerative disease.

Ecology: the study of an organism in relation to its environment.

Endocrine: the body's hormonal glands and system.

Endocrinology: study of the glands of internal secretion.

Enzyme: a protein substance that turns fuel into energy. Enzymes speed or control biological or chemical reactions in the body.

Erythrocytes: red blood cells containing haemoglobin. Main function is to transport oxygen.

Estrogen: female hormone produced by the ovaries.

Gastric: belonging to the stomach.

Gene: a factor that determines heredity.

Guillain-Barre syndrome: a form of swelling of the nerves which may develop between 1-3 weeks after a mild fever linked to a viral infection, or after immunisation. Pain and weakness affect the arms and legs and paralysis may develop. May last for weeks or months.

Hepatitis: inflammation of the liver; may be caused by bacterial or viral infections, chemicals, blood transfusions of infected blood. The liver can usually grow back its tissue, but severe hepatitis may lead to permanent damage. **Hepatitis A:** infectious hepatitis with slow onset. Usually followed by complete recovery. **Hepatitis B:** has rapid onset, may be severe and result in prolonged illness, carrier state, cirrhosis or liver cancer.

Histamine: a small protein molecule produced by mast cells throughout the body. Responsible for many of the symptoms of allergic response.

Hormone: a chemical substance produced in one part of the body that starts or runs activities in other parts of the body. Release of these hormones is regulated by other hormones, by nerve signals, and by signals from target organs indicating a decreased need for the stimulating hormone (the basic principle of oral and injected birth control agents).

Humoral mediated immunity: immune response generated by the fluids of the body.

Hypersensitivity: form of allergy generally mediated by antibodies.

Immune complexes: specific combinations of antibodies with their corresponding antigens.

Immune response: response of the body's immune system to antigens and allergens.

Immune tolerance: a state of non-responsiveness to a specific antigen.

Immunity: power to resist infection.

Immunoglobulin: any of 5 different antibodies (IgA, IgD, IgE, IgG, and IgM) formed in response to certain antigens.

IgA: secreted along mucous membranes, can neutralise invading viruses before they enter the body;

IgD: different from the others; functions not known.

IgE: important in triggering allergic reactions;

IgG: triggers immune responses: represents about 75% of the antibodies in the body; the only one which can cross the placental barrier – protects the foetus and the newborn infant from infection;

IgM: triggers immune responses.

Immunologic tolerance: specific suppression of immunity to antigens.

Immunology: the study of the reaction of the immune system to stimulation by antigens.

Leukopenia: an abnormal decrease in the number of white blood cells.

Lymph node: an organ of the immune system in which T cells and B cells are activated.

Lymphocyte: a type of white blood cell.

Macrophage: a large cell that cleans up debris in the bloodstream and activates other cells involved in immune response.

Mao: Monoamine oxidase, copper-containing enzyme which breaks down amines and is altered by the Pill. Used for depression and anxiety.

Mast cell: a cell found in tissues, esp. lungs and stomach, that releases histamines and other substances upon stimulation by irritants and allergens.

Mediate: to cause a change to occur (as stimulation by a hormone or foreign agent).

Metabolic disorder: any disorder that interferes with normal digestion, use of food and energy processes.

Metabolism: series of chemical processes in the living body by which life is maintained – relates to the movement of nutrients in the blood after digestion, resulting in growth, energy, release of wastes, and other body functions.

Microgram: one millionth of a gram.

Milligram: one thousandth of a gram.

Mitochondria: the part of a cell that provides it with its energy.

Monilia: thrush, a fungal infection.

Myasthenia gravis: condition of muscle wasting and weakness.

Natural killer cells (NK): special T cells which are the body's principal defence against renegade cells, e.g. cancer cells.

Neutropenia: an abnormal drop in the number of neutrophils (white blood cells) in the blood. Is linked to leukemia, infections, rheumatoid arthritis, vitamin B^{12} deficiency and a large spleen.

Normal flora: micro-organisms that live on or in the human body, and pose no health problems to immunocompetent individuals.

Nucleic acids: chemical compounds involved in making and storing energy, and carrying hereditary characteristics.

Nystatin: an anti-fungal antibiotic given to treat fungal infections of the digestive tract, vagina and skin. There are no known serious side effects though a few people are allergic to it.

Oophoritis: inflammation of the ovaries and fallopian tubes, now thought to be an autoimmune condition.

Opportunistic: micro-organisms that cause disease only when immune competency is lowered, e.g. candida albicans, toxoplasma gondii, and various viruses and fungi, salmonella and campylobacter varieties.

Parasympathetic nervous system: slows heart rate, increases intestinal and gland activity, relaxes ringlike muscles which close passages (sphincters); part of the autonomic nervous system.

Pathogen: a disease-causing micro-organism.

Pathology: branch of medicine that deals with changes in tissues or organs of the body causing or caused by disease.

Peripheral neuropathy: malfunction of nerves of the arms or legs.

Phagocyte: the 'big eater' cell (either macrophage or monocyte) that ingests other cells or debris.

Placebo: inactive substance given to a patient either for its pleasing effect or as a control in experiments with active drugs.

Porphyria: a disease caused by an enzyme dysfunction (usually in the liver), resulting in increased production of red pigments in the body with purplish urine, skin discolouration; also fatigue, depression, weakness. Usually hereditary, also caused by chemicals.

Raynaud's disease: chronic blood flow interruptions to the fingers, toes, ears and nose; become pale, then blush, then red. Also numbness, burning or pain. Often linked with conditions such as rheumatoid arthritis, protein defects, and CFS.

Retrovirus: unlike ordinary DNA viruses, retroviruses contain RNA as their genetic material. They integrate this into the genetic material of the cells they infect. There is dissension on the extent of their malignancy. They invariably mutate.

Reverse transcriptase: an enzyme carried by a retrovirus used to insert the viral gene into the normal cells. Laboratories can test the amount of this enzyme in blood or tissue.

RNA: ribonucleic acid; like DNA, an essential component of all living cells.

Sarcoma: non-cancerous tumour of muscle, bone, veins or other non-glandular tissue.

Serum sickness: when the body is overloaded with antigens (foreign molecules) and immune complexes form and are deposited in tissues. This causes inflammation in skin (urticaria), kidneys (albuminuria) and joints (arthritis).

SGOT: abbreviation for serum glutamic oxaloacetic transaminase, an enzyme found particularly in heart, liver and muscle tissue. A CFS marker: the body makes more of it when there has been some cell damage.

SGPT: abbreviation for serum glutamic pyruvic transaminase, an enzyme normally found in the liver. Having more of it than normal is a sign of liver damage.

SLE: systemic lupus erythematosus.

Staphylococcus: several types of bacteria; some are normally found in the body; others cause severe infections or produce toxins. Life-threatening staphylococcal infections can occur in association with high levels of candida or severely reduced immune competency.

Streptococcus: several types of pathogenic bacteria which can cause disease in almost any organ of the body.

Stress: basically any outside force or pressure on a living organism that causes atrophy in its normal physiological function.

Sympathetic nervous system: speeds up heart rate, narrows blood vessels and raises blood pressure; part of the autonomic nervous system.

Syndrome: a group of signs and symptoms that occur together and are typical of a particular disorder or disease.

Systemic lupus erythematosus: a chronic disease affecting many systems of the body. A butterfly rash on the face, weakness, fatigue and weight loss are the first symptoms. The skin may become sensitive to ultraviolet rays. Skin sores, loss of hair, suppurating mucosal membranes, kidney failue, severe nerve disorders, are among the most serious results of the disease.

T cells: Helper T cells: command the immune system, identify enemies, stimulate the production of killer T cells and antibodies.

Killer T cells: activated by helper T cells, they attack cancer cells and cells invaded by foreign bodies.

Suppressor T cells: slow down and stop the activities of B cells and other T cells. Important in switching off reactions when infections are conquered.

Thymus: a lymphatic gland in which T cells develop. It produces a zinc-dependent hormone called FTS which is needed for immunity.

Thyroiditis: inflammation of the thyroid gland; can be an auto-immune condition. Associated with thinning and brittle hair; brittle and ridged nails; pale, puffy and pasty complexion.

Toxoplasmosis: a parasitic infection carried by cats; has a most serious effect on the foetus, and on those with reduced immune competency.

Virus: a DNA or RNA genetic package that can grow only in the cells of another organism.

INDEX

2,4-D, 18

urinary tract infections, 117, 157
urinating, problems with, 95, 122
urine tests for allergies, 148
urine therapy, autoimmune, 150

vaccinations, 10
  side effects, 99, 123, 203
vaginal yeast infections, 107-8, 153-6
vertigo, 159
viruses, 31-8
  anti-viral agents, 170
  effects, 41-7, 57-8
  transmission, 39-40, 45-6
  types,
    arboviruses, 2, 44
    avian, 12
    Coxsackie, 2, 3, 6, 18, 19, 22, 46,
      101, 117
    cytomegalovirus, 44, 58
    Echo, 18, 44, 46
    enteroviruses, 44
    Epstein-Barr, 1, 7, 19, 31, 44, 45,
      46, 57
    hepatitis, 44, 46, 57
    herpesviruses, 6, 44, 50, 56, 57,
      122
    HHV6 (HBLV6), 6, 19, 45, 56, 57
    Human Immuno-deficiency
      (AIDS), 6, 49-50, 57, 64
    Marek's chicken, 45

  measles, 42, 44
  rubella, 44, 46
  smallpox, 99
  sub-acute-myelo-optico-
    neuropathy (SMON), 6
  vaccinia, 44
  varicella zoster, 44, 46
visual problems, 92, 110
visualisation, 65, 200
vitamin C, 95, 159, 163
vitamin E, 81, 155
vitiligo, 77
Voll, Reinholdt, 100
vomiting, 117

Walker, Morton, 80
water, 174, 197
weakness *see* strength, loss of
weaning, foods for, 203
Winbow, Adrian, 134
women's health problems 165-6 *see also
  under separate headings*
Wookey, Celia, 129
workplace, the, 196-7
Wraith, Derek, 69-70
Wright, Jonathon, 156

yoga, 37, 152, 192
yoghurt, 118, 155
Young, B.B., 131

zinc, 155, 170, 202

Lynne Alexander

Staying Vegetarian

Gourmet vegetarian cuisine, homemade yoghurt and fresh-baked bread, lettuce and strawberries straight from an organic garden and lovingly served, the pleasure of an imaginatively decorated home and gorgeous views, a warm and friendly welcome – such is the dream of vegetarians on the move or booking their holidays.

Lynne Alexander and her colleagues have stayed anonymously at over 80 guesthouses, hotels and B&Bs in England, Wales and Scotland, savouring their delights and eccentricities. Some are indeed the stuff of dreams, some leave much to be desired; whatever, *Staying Vegetarian* is honest, detailed, eloquent and practical in its assessment, a pleasure to read and a hawk-eyed guardian of vegetarian and vegan standards.

Uncommon Wisdom

Conversations with Remarkable People

Fritjof Capra

Fusing modern science and Eastern mysticism, Fritjof Capra took the intellectual world by storm with the publication of his hugely influential *The Tao of Physics*.

Now in *Uncommon Wisdom*, he charts the cultural, scientific and philosophical landmarks behind that intellectual odyssey through his conversations with some quite remarkable people: with Werner Heisenberg he explodes the myths of atomic physics, and searches for spiritual freedom alongside J. Krishnamurti; he pinpoints the nature of mental illness with R. D. Laing, and of ecological principles with E. F. Schumacher and Hazel Henderson, while Indira Gandhi stimulates his understanding of feminism in traditional Indian society.

All offer rich insight into the intellectual and artistic environment which helped shape one of this century's most fascinating world views of political, economic and social harmony.

'Remarkable . . . it causes the reader to do some hard thinking on his own. *Uncommon Wisdom* is certainly worth reading' Frederik Pohl, *New Scientist*

'In the role of interpreter of the "philosophy" of physics today, Dr Capra has few equals' John Gribbin, *Times Educational Supplement*

FONTANA PAPERBACKS

The Successful Self
Freeing our Hidden Inner Strengths
Dorothy Rowe

Is it possible to be truly successful as a person? Or must we, as most of us do, continue to live our lives feeling in some way trapped and oppressed, frustrated, irritable, haunted by worries and regrets, creating misery for ourselves and others?

In *The Successful Self* leading psychologist Dorothy Rowe, author of *Beyond Fear*, shows us how to live more comfortably and creatively within ourselves by achieving a fuller understanding of how we experience our existence and how we perceive the threat of its annihilation.

She demonstrates how to develop the social and personal skills we lack, retaining the uniqueness of our individuality while becoming an integral part of the life around us and learning how to value and accept ourselves.

With characteristic originality, clarity and unfailing wisdom, Dorothy Rowe enables us to revolutionise our own lives and the lives of others in the process of becoming a Successful Self.

'Dorothy Rowe stands out amongst psychologists for her clear insight into human experience: her writing is refreshingly free from the dubious theoretical constructs and jargon ideas which plague this subject' Oliver Gillie, *Independent*

'A very brightly written book that intriguingly makes you question something most of us discuss: do we really like ourselves? Then it goes on to help us do so' Mavis Nicholson

A FONTANA ORIGINAL